T0229062

Head and Neck Ultrasound

Guest Editors

JOSEPH C. SNIEZEK, MD
ROBERT A. SOFFERMAN, MD

ULTRASOUND CLINICS

www.ultrasound.theclinics.com

Consulting Editor
VIKRAM DOGRA, MD

April 2012 • Volume 7 • Number 2

SAUNDERS an imprint of ELSEVIER, Inc.

W.B. SAUNDERS COMPANY
A Division of Elsevier Inc.

1600 John F. Kennedy Boulevard ● Suite 1800 ● Philadelphia, Pennsylvania 19103-2899

http://www.theclinics.com

ULTRASOUND CLINICS Volume 7, Number 2
April 2012 ISSN 1556-858X, ISBN-13: 978-1-4557-4223-3

Editor: Donald Mumford

Ultrasound Clinics (ISSN 1556-858X) is published quarterly by W.B. Saunders, 360 Park Avenue South, New York, NY 10010-1710. Months of publication are January, April, July, and October. Business and editorial offices: 1600 John F. Kennedy Boulevard, Suite 1800, Philadelphia, Pennsylvania 19103-2899. Accounting and circulation offices: 6277 Sea Harbor Drive, Orlando, FL 32887-4800. Periodicals postage paid at New York, NY, and additional mailing offices. Subscription prices are $243 per year for (US individuals), $297 per year for (US institutions), $139 per year for (US students and residents), $273 per year for (Canadian individuals), $332 per year for (Canadian institutions), $291 per year for (international individuals), $332 per year for (international institutions), and $139 per year for (Canadian and foreign students/residents). To receive student/resident rate, orders must be accompanied by name of affiliated institution, date of term, and the signature of program/residency coordinator on institution letterhead. Orders will be billed at individual rate until proof of status is received. Foreign air speed delivery is included in all Clinics subscription prices. All prices are subject to change without notice. **POSTMASTER:** Send address changes to *Ultrasound Clinics,* Elsevier Health Sciences Division, Subscription Customer Service, 3251 Riverport Lane, Maryland Heights, MO 63043. **Customer Service (orders, claims, online, change of address): Telephone: 1-800-654-2452 (U.S. and Canada); 314-447-8871 (outside U.S. and Canada). Fax: 314-447-8029. E-mail: journalscustomerservice-usa@elsevier.com (for print support); journalsonlinesupport-usa@elsevier.com (for online support).**

Reprints: For copies of 100 or more, of articles in this publication, please contact the Commercial Reprints Department, Elsevier Inc., 360 Park Avenue South, New York, NY 10010-1710. Tel.: (+1) 212-633-3812; Fax: (+1) 212-462-1935; E-mail: reprints@elsevier.com.

Printed in the United States of America.

Transferred to Digital Printing, 2012

Contributors

CONSULTING EDITOR

VIKRAM DOGRA, MD
Professor of Radiology, Urology, and
Biomedical Engineering, Director of Ultrasound
and Associate Chair for Education and
Research, Department of Imaging Sciences,
University of Rochester School of Medicine
and Dentistry, Rochester, New York

GUEST EDITORS

JOSEPH C. SNIEZEK, MD
Otolaryngology/Head & Neck Surgery,
Tripler Army Medical Center, MCHK-DSH;
Department of Surgery, John A. Burns School
of Medicine, University of Hawaii,
Honolulu, Hawaii

ROBERT A. SOFFERMAN, MD
Division of Otolaryngology, University of
Vermont School of Medicine, Fletcher Allen
Health Care, Burlington, Vermont

AUTHORS

JEFFREY M. BUMPOUS, MD
Department of Surgery, University of Louisville,
University Surgical Associates, Louisville,
Kentucky

BENJAMIN B. CABLE, MD
Uniformed Services University of the Health
Sciences, Bethesda, Maryland; Pediatric
Otolaryngology/Head & Neck Surgery,
Tripler Army Medical Center,
Honolulu, Hawaii

JAMES S. GREEN, MBBS, FRCA
Department of Anesthesiology and Pain
Medicine, University of Alberta, Edmonton,
Alberta, Canada

MICHAEL R. HOLTEL, MD
Telemedicine Research Institute, University
of Hawaii, Honolulu, Hawaii; Telemedicine and
Advanced Technology Research Center of the
United States Army Medical Readiness and
Materiel Command, Ft Detrick, Maryland

GERALD T. KANGELARIS, MD
Department of Otolaryngology – Head & Neck
Surgery, University of California,
San Francisco, San Francisco, California

THERESA B. KIM, MD
Department of Otolaryngology – Head & Neck
Surgery, University of California, San
Francisco, San Francisco, California;
Department of Otolaryngology, Pediatric
Otolaryngology, St Louis, Missouri

CHRISTOPHER KLEM, MD
Otolaryngology–Head and Neck Surgery
Service, Tripler Army Medical Center,
Honolulu, Hawaii

LISA LEE, MD
Department of Otolaryngology–Head and Neck
Surgery, University of Cincinnati Medical
Center, Medical Sciences Building,
Cincinnati, Ohio

THOMAS MAILHOT, MD, RDMS
Department of Emergency Medicine,
Los Angeles County + USC Medical Center,
General Hospital, Los Angeles, California

DIKU MANDAVIA, MD, FACEP, FRCPC
LA County + USC Medical Center, Department
of Emergency Medicine, Cedars-Sinai Medical
Center, Department of Emergency Medicine,
General Hospital, Los Angeles, California

LISA A. ORLOFF, MD
Department of Otolaryngology–Head & Neck
Surgery, University of California,
San Francisco, San Francisco, California

PHILLIPS PERERA, MD, RDMS, FACEP
Department of Emergency Medicine,
Los Angeles County + USC Medical Center,
General Hospital, Los Angeles, California

GREGORY W. RANDOLPH, MD
Massachusetts Eye and Ear Infirmary, Boston,
Massachusetts

DAVID RILEY, MD, MS, RDMS, RDCS, RVT
Division of Emergency Medicine, New York
Presbyterian Hospital, Columbia University
Medical Center, New York, New York

VERONICA J. ROOKS, MD
Uniformed Services University of the Health
Sciences, Bethesda, Maryland; Pediatric
Radiology, Department of Radiology, Tripler
Army Medical Center, Honolulu, Hawaii

RUSSELL B. SMITH, MD
Department of Otolaryngology—Head and
Neck Surgery, Nebraska Methodist Estabrook
Cancer Center, Omaha, Nebraska

ROBERT A. SOFFERMAN, MD
Division of Otolaryngology, University of
Vermont School of Medicine, Fletcher Allen
Health Care, Burlington, Vermont

DAVID L. STEWARD, MD
Department of Otolaryngology–Head and Neck
Surgery, University of Cincinnati Medical
Center, Medical Sciences Building,
Cincinnati, Ohio

BAN C.H. TSUI, MD, FRCPC
Department of Anesthesiology and Pain
Medicine, University of Alberta, Edmonton,
Alberta, Canada

Contents

parathyroidectomy. In conjunction with functional sestamibi scanning, ultrasonography permits accurate localization of enlarged parathyroid glands in the vast majority of patients with hyperparathyroidism. Consequently, ultrasound technology applied to parathyroid pathology facilitates directed surgical therapy and minimally invasive applications. As such, ultrasonography holds great promise as a tool that enables cost-effective and advanced patient care.

Ultrasound-Guided Procedures for the Office

Russell B. Smith

Ultrasonography has an ever increasing role in the management of a wide variety of diseases affecting the head and neck. While ultrasonography is most commonly used for imaging of thyroid pathology, it also can be utilized in a host of diagnostic and therapeutic procedures. This article reviews the office-based ultrasound-guided procedures in the head and neck and discusses technical considerations for performing these interventions. Video versions of several figures in this article can be viewed at www.ultrasound.theclinics.com.

Head and Neck Ultrasound in the Pediatric Population

Veronica J. Rooks and Benjamin B. Cable

Ultrasound, as a diagnostic modality, has been developing rapidly. High-resolution ultrasound machines have been reduced to the size of a laptop computer. Ultrasound can be adopted by otolaryngologists for use within the clinic and the operating room. Ultrasound offers several advantages to the pediatric patient population. It is well tolerated and adds a degree of precision to the physical examination. It can be done repeatedly as lesions evolve and treatment is performed. It is valuable for guidance and therapeutic treatment of lesions in the operating room. It is likely that ultrasound use will continue to rapidly grow and evolve as a tool within the field of otolaryngology.

Emerging Technology in Head and Neck Ultrasonography

Michael R. Holtel

Increased use of ultrasonography of the head and neck by clinicians has resulted from more compact, higher resolution ultrasound machines that can be more readily used in the office setting. Palm-sized machines are already used for vascular access and bladder assessment. As the resolution of these machines becomes adequate for head and neck assessment, ultrasonography is likely to become a routine adjunct to the office physical examination. Further techniques to reduce artifact beyond spatial compounding, second harmonics, and broadband inversion techniques are likely to be developed to improve ultrasound images. Manual palpation using the ultrasound transducer or "sound palpation," using sound to recreate vibration provides information on tissue "stiffness," which has been successfully used to distinguish between benign and malignant lesions in the head and neck (particularly thyroid nodules). Microbubble contrast-enhanced ultrasound provides improved resolution of ultrasound images. Three- and four-dimensional ultrasonography provides for more accurate diagnosis. The ability of microbubbles with ligands affixed to their outer surface to target specific tissue makes them excellent delivery vehicles. DNA plasmids, chemotherapy agents, and therapeutic drugs can be released at a specific anatomic site. The motion of microbubbles stimulated by ultrasound can be used to increase drug penetration through tissues and has been shown to be effective in breaking up clots in stroke patients (without increased risk). High-intensity focused ultrasound can be used to create coagulation necrosis without significant damage to adjacent tissue. It has been effectively used in neurosurgery and urology, but its effectiveness in the head and neck is still being determined. A prototype for surgical navigation with ultrasound has been developed for the head and neck, which allows real-time imaging of anatomic surgical changes.

This article presents a comprehensive narrative review of the published literature relating to ultrasound imaging relevant to anesthesia for ear, nose, and throat (ENT) surgery. The review comprises 2 main subject areas: the use of ultrasonography related to assessment and management of the airway, and the use of ultrasonography related to nerve blockade for ENT surgery. The relevant sonoanatomy and suitable probe placement are illustrated in relation to applicable regional anatomy (they are not discussed). The possible value of the use of ultrasonography to improve existing clinical practice in these areas is explored.

Special Article in Emergency Ultrasound

The RUSH exam (Rapid Ultrasound in SHock examination), presented in this article, represents a comprehensive algorithm for the integration of bedside ultrasound into the care of the patient in shock. By focusing on a stepwise evaluation of the shock patient defined here as "Pump, Tank, and Pipes," clinicians will gain crucial anatomic and physiologic data to better care for these patients. Video versions for many of this article's figures can be viewed at www.ultrasound.theclinics.com.

Ultrasound Clinics

THE CLINICS ARE NOW AVAILABLE ONLINE!

Access your subscription at:
www.theclinics.com

Foreword

It is my pleasure to introduce this new issue of *Ultrasound Clinics* dedicated to the utility of ultrasound in the evaluation of head and neck diseases. With growing concerns for radiation exposure, the use of high-frequency ultrasound has increased in the recent times. Ultrasound allows real-time imaging of soft tissues of the neck, thyroid gland, parathyroid glands, and lymph node characterization. In addition, ultrasound is also used for fine-needle aspiration biopsy of thyroid masses and other soft tissue lesions.

This issue of *Ultrasound Clinics* covers normal anatomy and provides a succinct overview of diseases involving the head and neck. Important pearls and pitfalls needed by radiology residents, practicing radiologists, and surgeons are highlighted in this issue. An article for parathyroid localization and thyroid disease evaluation is included. Other topics of interest in this issue are ultrasound-guided procedures, emerging technologies in ultrasound for head and neck applications, and an approach to the interpretation of head and neck ultrasound.

I want to thank our contributors for their outstanding work.

With best wishes,

Vikram Dogra, MD
Department of Imaging Sciences
University of Rochester Medical Center
601 Elmwood Avenue, Box 648
Rochester, NY 14642-8648, USA

E-mail address:
Vikram_Dogra@URMC.Rochester.edu

Ultrasound Clin 7 (2012) xi
doi:10.1016/j.cult.2012.01.001
1556-858X/12/$ – see front matter

Head and Neck Anatomy and Ultrasound Correlation

Christopher Klem, MD

KEYWORDS

• Ultrasound • Head and neck • Normal anatomy

ULTRASOUND OF HEAD AND NECK: ANATOMY

Ultrasonography of the head and neck has been performed for decades, primarily by radiologists. Recent improvements in high-resolution ultrasound have made the technology much more accessible to clinicians. Office-based ultrasound allows clinicians to personally perform a real-time diagnostic radiographic procedure and literally see pathology below the skin. This ability makes ultrasound an important extension of the physical examination and enables clinicians to more rapidly and effectively treat patients.

A thorough knowledge of the complex anatomy of the head and neck is essential to understanding the ultrasonographic appearance of this region. The frequent performance of surgical procedures leads to a familiarity with anatomic structures that makes active radiographic imaging like ultrasound especially suited for use by surgeons. It is important to understand and appreciate the normal sonographic appearance of head and neck structures before recognizing abnormal pathology.

An ultrasound examination should follow a systematic and thorough course to ensure that all structures of the neck from clavicle to mandible are evaluated. The examination is usually performed in both the axial and longitudinal planes. In gaining experience, a beginning ultrasonographer typically develops a structured routine that ultimately leads to a comprehensive, yet expeditious, sonographic evaluation.

An appreciation of the basic physics and principles of ultrasound is important to be able to recognize the central characteristics of various tissue types. The sonographic appearance of fat is hyperechoic relative to muscle, which is hypoechoic. The cervical fascia that invests the muscles and organs of the neck is very echogenic and is seen clearly as a distinct white line that delineates structures from one another. Mucosa is also very echogenic and can be easily differentiated from the hypoechoic muscle that it typically overlies. Arteries are anechoic and pulsations can often be seen. Veins are also anechoic and easily compressible with pressure from the ultrasound probe.

Division of the neck into anatomic triangles based on the sternocleidomastoid, digastric, and omohyoid muscles, all of which are readily identified sonographically, creates easily recognizable landmarks on which to base a thorough examination. These triangles do not correspond exactly with the American Joint Committee on Cancer levels of the neck for cancer staging, but an examiner may do simple correlations using sonographic landmarks.[1]

The triangular-shaped area anterior to the sternocleidomastoid muscle is anatomically classified as the anterior triangle, whereas the region posterior to the muscle is termed the posterior triangle. The anterior triangle is further divided into infrahyoid and suprahyoid sections. The anterior belly of the digastric muscle subdivides the suprahyoid portion into the submandibular triangle posteriorly

This article was previously published in the December 2010 issue of *Otolaryngologic Clinics of North America*.
Otolaryngology – Head and Neck Surgery Service, Tripler Army Medical Center, 1 Jarrett White Road, Honolulu, HI 96859-5000, USA
E-mail address: christopher.klem@us.army.mil

Ultrasound Clin 7 (2012) 161–166
doi:10.1016/j.cult.2011.12.001

and submental triangle anteriorly. Below the posterior belly of the digastric muscle, the infrahyoid triangle is divided into the muscular and carotid triangles by the superior belly of the omohyoid muscle.

Borders of the posterior triangle include the sternocleidomastoid muscle anteriorly, the occiput superiorly, the clavicle inferiorly, and the trapezius muscle posteriorly. The inferior belly of the omohyoid muscle subdivides the region into the occipital triangle superiorly and the supraclavicular triangle inferiorly.

SUBMENTAL TRIANGLE (LEVEL 1A)

The anterior bellies of the right and left digastric muscles form the lateral borders of the submental triangle. The apex of the triangle is the mental symphysis, the base is the hyoid bone, and the mylohyoid muscle forms the floor. Lymph nodes are the only structures of note that reside in the submental space.

Visible via transverse imaging through the submental region are the extrinsic muscles of the tongue, including the genioglossus, geniohyoid, and hyoglossus muscles (**Fig. 1**). The sling-shaped mylohyoid muscle forms the floor of the mouth.

The lingual artery courses medial to the hyoglossus muscle, whereas the submandibular duct runs alongside the sublingual gland between the hyoglossus and more superficial mylohyoid muscle. These muscles are readily distinguished from

one another, and the hyoglossus muscle can be seen contracting when the patient's tongue is moved from side to side during active ultrasonography, whereas the mylohyoid remains immobile. The hyperechoic sublingual gland is elongated and fills much of the lateral floor of mouth extending posteriorly from the submandibular gland toward the mental symphysis anteriorly.[2] An abnormally dilated submandibular duct is easily seen sonographically in the floor of the mouth, but a normal duct is less evident. The duct is differentiated from the lingual artery and vein by the lack of flow on Doppler imaging.

SUBMANDIBULAR TRIANGLE (LEVEL 1B)

The submandibular triangle is bounded by the anterior and posterior digastric bellies inferiorly and the mandible superiorly. Forming the medial border of this triangle are the hyoglossus and mylohyoid muscles. The sublingual space lies deep to the mylohyoid muscle (**Fig. 2**). The mylohyoid muscle is the key to determining whether or not pathology resides in the sublingual or submandibular space; a lesion deep to the mylohyoid arises from the sublingual space, whereas anything superficial to the muscle rests in the submandibular space.

Normal submandibular gland is homogenous and hyperechoic compared with surrounding structures.[3,4] There are also lymph nodes and fat that reside in the submandibular space, but unlike

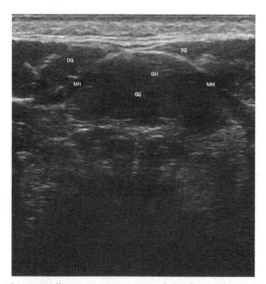

Fig. 1. Midline transverse view of the floor of mouth and tongue from the submental region. Clearly seen are the paired anterior digastric muscles (DG) and mylohyoid muscles (MH), as well as the genioglossus (GG) and geniohyoid muscles (GH).

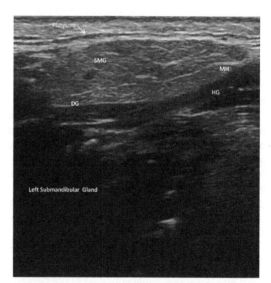

Fig. 2. The homogenous echogenicity of the submandibular gland (SMG) is clearly seen in the transverse view, along with surrounding structures, including the anterior digastric muscle (DG), mylohyoid muscle (MH), hyoglossus muscle (HG), and platysma.

the parotid gland, there are no lymph nodes within the submandibular gland parenchyma. Any sonographic abnormalities in the gland should be considered pathologic. Because the sonographic characteristics of nerve are so similar to the surrounding tissue, the hypoglossal and lingual nerves are not usually visible.

The facial artery is a key feature of the submandibular space and is easily followed on its circuitous course from the external carotid artery through the triangle to the point where it crosses the body of the mandible. More superficially, the anterior facial vein and retromandibular vein are readily visualized. The retromandibular vein is an excellent landmark for distinguishing parotid space pathology posteriorly from submandibular gland disease anteriorly.[2] Wharton's duct is often visible when dilated due to distal obstruction, but a normal duct is not commonly seen.

CAROTID TRIANGLE/MUSCULAR TRIANGLE (LEVELS 2, 3, 4)

Inferior to the posterior belly of the digastric is the carotid triangle, bounded anteriorly by the superior belly of the omohyoid muscle and posteriorly by the sternocleidomastoid muscle.

Immediately evident sonographically are the vascular structures of the carotid sheath, including the carotid artery and internal jugular vein. Especially in this region, color flow Doppler helps distinguish blood vessels from other structures. It is important to scan in both the axial and longitudinal planes because blood vessels are round when the transducer is axial and appear as an anechoic linear structure when the transducer is longitudinal (Fig. 3). The vagus nerve can sometimes be seen as a dot on axial imaging or as a hypoechoic line medial to the carotid artery on longitudinal imaging (Fig. 4A).[5]

The internal jugular vein is typically lateral and slightly superficial to the artery. There is variability in the size of the vein, with the right side typically larger than the left. The vein is easily compressible with gentle pressure from the ultrasound transducer, whereas the carotid artery is not. When a patient performs a Valsalva maneuver, the vein also dilates (see Fig. 4).

More superiorly in this region, the internal and external carotid arteries, as well as the bifurcation of the artery, are readily seen deep and anterior to the hypoechoic sternocleidomastoid muscle. Unlike the compressible internal jugular vein, the carotid artery is pulsatile and does not compress easily or change size with Valsalva. Also common is a posterior enhancement effect, an artifact that is present when the distal reflected echoes behind an area of low attenuation (in this case, anechoic blood in the lumen of the carotid artery) appear enhanced compared with adjacent tissue. External carotid branches can often be followed distally from their origin. The carotid bifurcation is at approximately the level of the hyoid bone and marks the lower limit of level 2.

Scanning inferiorly from the carotid bifurcation, the common carotid artery, internal jugular vein, and sternocleidomastoid muscle are the major structures in the field of view. The inferior border of level 3 and the carotid triangle is the superior belly of the omohyoid muscle, a hypoechoic structure that runs obliquely from posteroinferior to anterosuperior across the superficial aspect of the internal jugular vein.

Lymph nodes are commonly seen in the carotid and muscular triangles. Nonpathologic lymph nodes are oval or kidney bean shaped, hypoechoic, and have a central fatty hilum that is echogenic

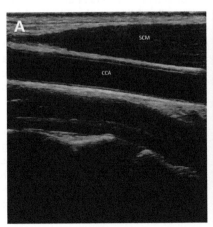
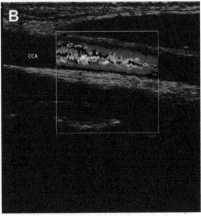

Fig. 3. Longitudinal view of the common carotid artery (CCA) and sternocleidomastoid muscle (SCM) (A). Color flow Doppler in the sagittal plane confirms that a structure is vascular in nature (B).

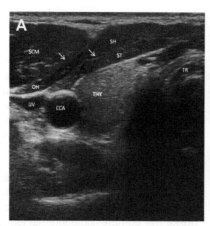
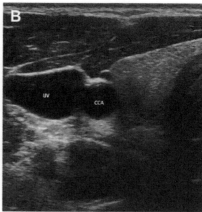

Fig. 4. Transverse image of the right thyroid lobe. Note the compressed internal jugular vein (IJV) lateral to the common carotid artery (CCA) (*A*) compared with the distended internal jugular vein (*B*) when the patient performs a Valsalva maneuver. Also well seen are the thyroid gland (THY), tracheal rings (TR), the sternocleidomastoid muscle (SCM), and the omohyoid (OH), sternohyoid (SH), and sternothyroid (ST) muscles all separated by a fascial layer (*arrows*).

(**Fig. 5**). Running through the hilum are afferent and efferent lymphatics as well as arterial and venous supply that can often be seen on color flow Doppler. The size criteria for what is considered a pathologic lymph node is controversial; many use 1.0 cm as the upper limit of normal for otherwise ordinary-appearing lymph nodes, except for the jugulodigastric node, which is given an upper limit of 1.5 cm. Regardless of size, in the presence of a known malignancy, a lymph node without a normal sonographic appearance should be considered suspicious for metastatic spread.

The muscular triangle, which corresponds to level 4, is bordered superiorly by the superior belly of the omohyoid, posteriorly by the sternocleidomastoid muscle, and anteriorly by the sternohyoid muscle. Carotid sheath structures, the anterior scalene muscle, and lymphatics are the prevalent structures in the muscular triangle. This muscle originates from the transverse processes of the cervical spine, runs deep to the carotid sheath, and attaches to the first rib. Inferiorly, the common carotid artery can be followed to its junction with the subclavian artery by aiming the transducer cephalad.

POSTERIOR TRIANGLE (LEVEL 5)

Initially, the posterior triangle can be a challenging region to understand sonographically. The region is superficial and is comprised primarily of muscles around the border and the floor. Forming the deep boundary of the triangle are the scalene, levator scapulae, and splenius capitis muscles. The inferior belly of the omohyoid muscle delineates the occipital triangle above from the supraclavicular triangle below. Residing in the cervical fascia superficial to the floor are the spinal accessory nerve and lymph nodes, fat, the brachial plexus, and the transverse cervical artery and vein. The spinal accessory nerve is difficult to see on ultrasound.

Inferior to the inferior belly of the omohyoid muscle, the supraclavicular triangle is also bounded by the trapezius muscle posteriorly, the sternocleidomastoid muscle anteriorly, and the clavicle inferiorly. The subclavian vein is often seen posterior to the clavicle. Emerging from the lateral aspect of the scalene muscles, the brachial plexus can be seen as rounded hypoechoic structures on axial imaging.

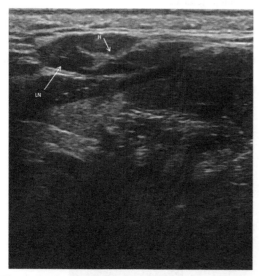

Fig. 5. Benign lymph node. Note the oblong, hypoechoic nature of the lymph node (LN) and the hyperechoic, fatty hilum (H) that includes the vascular pedicle (*arrows*).

THYROID/PARATHYROID

High-resolution ultrasound of the thyroid gland reveals remarkable detail about the gland and surrounding structures. Coupled with the superficial location in the anterior neck, this is an excellent region for beginning ultrasonographers to gain experience and confidence.

Normal thyroid parenchyma is hyperechoic and homogenous compared with the relatively hypoechoic strap muscles, the sternothyroid and sternohyoid, that border the gland anteriorly. The cervical fascia investing the muscles and the thyroid gland is echogenic and appears as a thin white line (see **Fig. 4**). Interruption of the fascia surrounding the gland should alert an examiner to the possibility of extrathyroidal extension by a malignancy.

There is commonly slight asymmetry between the right and left thyroid lobes, both in size and location. Although present in approximately 80% of people, the pyramidal lobe is not commonly seen because of its small diameter.

The trachea lies posterior to the thyroid and the common carotid arteries border the gland laterally on each side. The esophagus is typically seen inferiorly, deep to the left thyroid lobe.

Both the superior and inferior thyroid arteries can be traced from their origins at the external carotid artery and thyrocervical trunk, respectively, to the gland. The inferior thyroid artery passes deep to the common carotid artery and where the vessel enters the gland is an excellent marker for the depth of the recurrent laryngeal nerve. Color flow Doppler is essential to aid in differentiating blood vessels from cystic thyroid pathology.

Ultrasound evaluation for parathyroids is usually done as a localization study preoperatively in the setting of primary hyperparathyroidism. Normal parathyroid glands are rarely visible sonographically. The superior glands are more predictably found in close proximity to the cricothyroid joint, whereas the inferior glands have a more variable location.

LARYNX/TRACHEA/ESOPHAGUS (LEVEL 6)

Despite being air filled, the structures of the larynx and trachea lie superficially in the neck and have good inherent soft tissue contrast making them ideally suited for visualization with ultrasound.

In the midline of the neck deep to the thyroid gland, the cartilaginous tracheal rings and cricoid are useful landmarks in both the axial and longitudinal planes (**Fig. 6**). The cricoid cartilage forms a complete ring and is the most cephalad portion of the trachea. Below the cricoid, the first 5 to 6 tracheal rings can be seen with gentle neck extension. Several reports of the use of high-resolution

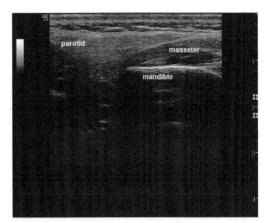

Fig. 6. Parotid gland.

ultrasound to assist with visualization of the trachea during percutaneous tracheotomy are published.[6,7]

The larynx lies between the cricoid cartilage inferiorly and the hyoid bone superiorly. Variable ossification of the laryngeal framework, including the thyroid and cricoid cartilages, causes the sonographic appearance of the larynx to differ significantly between patients. The thyroid, cricoid, and arytenoid cartilages are all echogenic, whereas the intrinsic muscles of the larynx appear hypoechoic. The laryngeal mucosa is also hyperechoic, in contrast to the anechoic intraluminal air column. The differing acoustic characteristics allow differentiation of these structures. Fat in the pre-epiglottic space is echogenic, whereas the

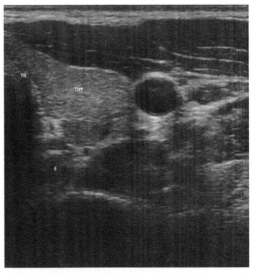

Fig. 7. In the lower neck, the esophagus (E) is typically seen on the left side adjacent to the trachea (TR) and deep to the left thyroid lobe (THY).

cartilage of the epiglottis is hypoechoic. This region is best visualized via the thyrohyoid membrane.[5]

Usually to the left of the trachea, the esophagus has a characteristic echogenic center of air and saliva with a hypoechoic muscular rim, often described as a bull's eye or target (**Fig. 7**). When a patient swallows, the hyperechoic esophageal center dilates actively and then returns to the resting state.[2]

PAROTID SPACE

The boundaries of the parotid space are the external auditory canal superiorly, the masseter muscle anteriorly, and the mandible and medial pterygoid muscle medially. The posterior digastric muscle is the inferior border of the parotid space and forms the superior boundary of the carotid triangle below.[5]

Normal parotid tissue is sonographically similar to submandibular gland and is hyperechoic and homogenous. When scanning, areas in the gland that are hypoechoic suggest abnormal pathology.[8]

Multiple lymph nodes normally reside in the gland and may be evident on ultrasound examination. Although the facial nerve itself is not visible sonographically, the retromandibular vein travels in a craniocaudad direction and its location is a reliable approximation for the depth of the facial nerve (see **Fig. 6**). Arbitrary delineation of superficial and deep lobes of the parotid gland can be made with the retromandibular vein as the reference. Although a dilated parotid (Stensen's) duct is readily sonographically apparent, a normal duct can sometimes be seen as an echogenic line within the superficial lobe. When an accessory parotid lobe is present, it typically lies along the course of the parotid duct lateral to the masseter muscle.[2]

ANATOMY KNOWLEDGE ESSENTIAL FOR EFFECTIVE ULTRASOUND

Ultrasound is an effective instrument for otolaryngology–head and neck surgeons. A thorough knowledge of head and neck anatomy, as well as the sonographic appearance of normal anatomic structures in this complex region, is essential. The comprehensive familiarity with head and neck anatomy gained through surgery makes ultrasound especially suited to use by surgeons.

REFERENCES

1. Agur AM. Grant's atlas of anatomy. 12th edition. Baltimore (MD): Williams & Wilkins; 2008.
2. Evans RM. Anatomy and technique. In: Ahuja A, Evans R, editors. Practical head and neck ultrasound. London: Greenwich Medical Media Ltd; 2003. p. 1–16.
3. Alyas F, Lewis K, Williams M, et al. Diseases of the submandibular gland as demonstrated using high resolution ultrasound. Br J Radiol 2005;78:362–9.
4. Howlett DC, Alyas F, Wong KT, et al. Sonographic assessment of the submandibular space. Clin Radiol 2004;59:1070–8.
5. Gourin CG, Orlorr LA. Normal head and neck ultrasound anatomy. In: Orloff LA, editor. Head and neck ultrasonography. San Diego (CA): Plural Publishing Inc; 2008. p. 39–68.
6. Bertram S, Emshoff R, Norer B. Ultrasonographic anatomy of the anterior neck: Implications for tracheostomy. J Oral Maxillofac Surg 1995;53:1420–4.
7. Muhammad JK, Patton DW, Evans RM, et al. Percutaneous dilational tracheostomy (PDT) under ultrasound guidance. Br J Oral Maxillofac Surg 1999;37:309–11.
8. Zajkowski P, Jakubowski W, Bialek EJ, et al. Pleomorphic adenoma and adenolymphoma in ultrasonography. Eur J Ultrasound 2000;12:23–9.

Interpretation of Ultrasound

Robert A. Sofferman, MD

KEYWORDS

- Ultrasound interpretation • Pathologic correlation
- Sonographic artifacts • Head and neck ultrasonography

A thorough knowledge of head and neck anatomy is critical to defining what are normal and abnormal findings on high-resolution ultrasound. At first, the transverse and sagittal orientations of the transducer can be confusing to the operator. The best way to overcome this problem is to select concentrated areas of the neck and identify as many normal structures as possible within that area. Instead of using a Doppler whenever a suspect blood vessel is identified, the operator will better understand relationships by tracing as much as possible the course of the vessel in gray scale both in transverse and sagittal planes. The transition from normal anatomy and a sound knowledge of scanning artifacts will serve as the best foundation for properly interpreting pathologic conditions.

ULTRASOUND INTERPRETATION IN HEAD AND NECK PATHOLOGY

The beauty of ultrasound is that the examination process occurs in real time with the examiner learning how to merge the various planes of view into a dynamic 3-dimensional image. There is no substitute for the circumstance where the operator/managing clinician is performing this dynamic examination while constructing a concurrent differential diagnosis. A technician who does not possess the knowledge base of head and neck pathology is quite limited in this aspect of ultrasonography. However, radiologic technicians and radiologists are well educated about standardizing the examination process. This redundancy from one examination to the next is valuable in comparison of normal with abnormal structure, and it lessens the likelihood of omissions.

The otolaryngologist who performs office-based ultrasound must avoid cutting corners in defense of time to maintain a proper standard and to avoid overlooking a key portion of the examination. As an example, it is easy to omit a proper survey of lymph node basins when concentrating on a thyroid nodule and, of course, both elements may be linked and are important to examine in the same ultrasound procedure. Conversely, a thyroid examination should be part of every head and neck ultrasound procedure. Thyroid pathology is common and malignancies can be occult and asymptomatic. In a similar manner, lymphadenopathy alone may not be as meaningful as lymphadenopathy in conjunction with an irregular thyroid nodule containing microcalcifications.

This article is constructed to present some of the pathologic conditions that affect the salivary glands, soft tissues, lymph nodes, thyroid and parathyroid glands, esophagus, vascular structures, congenital cysts, and even mandibular relationships. The content provides the physician with information and representative images of the more common conditions involving the head and neck. Some of this information may also be covered elsewhere in this publication, but it is presented here as a systems overview and stepping point for further in-depth study. High-resolution ultrasound is the best modality for detailing pathology of the thyroid gland before fine-needle aspiration cytology. An enlarged

This article was previously published in the December 2010 issue of *Otolaryngologic Clinics of North America*.
Division of Otolaryngology, University of Vermont School of Medicine, Fletcher Allen Health Care, ACC West Pavilion 4th Floor, 111 Colchester Avenue, Burlington, VT 05401, USA
E-mail address: robert.sofferman@vtmednet.org

Ultrasound Clin 7 (2012) 167–190
doi:10.1016/j.cult.2011.12.002

ultrasound.theclinics.com

parotid gland is often mystifying at initial history and physical examination, but the added advantage of concurrent ultrasound usually allows the clinician to understand the problem and direct earlier proper management.

Skin and Subcutaneous Tissues

High-resolution transducers in the range of 10 to 12 MHz provide good detail of the skin and subcutaneous tissues. If one has access to even higher frequency probes, ie, 17 MHz, the image detail can be stunning. One very helpful use of the ultrasound examination of a skin-related process is to differentiate cellulitis from abscess, especially in children. A cellulitic process is diffuse and edema of the tissues can be identified on ultrasound. In contrast, an abscess is usually a discrete hypoechoic to anechoic area that may extend deep to the subcutaneous plane (**Fig. 1**). A foreign body can usually be identified even if it is not ferromagnetic or may not demonstrate on conventional soft tissue radiograph. Fistulous tracts are hypoechoic channels that usually can be traced to the site of origin (**Fig. 2**). If the fistula arises from the skin surface, the tract can be easily traced and the condition properly identified. A fistula arising from the aerodigestive tract that extends into the subcutaneous tissues or thyroid (fourth branchial pouch sinus) may be traceable on ultrasound (**Fig. 3**).

Frequently, ultrasound is the initial study as part of a more comprehensive imaging profile. In many instances, it can suffice as the only requisite study. A sebaceous cyst is usually properly identified and characterized by physical examination alone, but it is instructive to demonstrate its sonographic characteristics (**Fig. 4**A, B). It is usually seen at the level

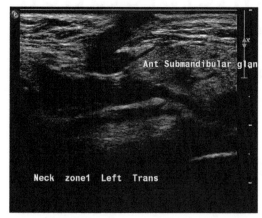

Fig. 2. A fistula from the mandible to submandibular skin is associated in this circumstance with a prior dental implant.

of the dermis and can extend by pressure enlargement to involve the subcutaneous level. The mass is discrete and well-encapsulated and the contained sebum does not produce as homogeneous an image as a fluid-filled cyst. Posterior enhancement is present to some degree. Lipomas are common and usually arise from the subcutaneous adipose tissues (**Fig. 5**A). They have a soft, somewhat compressible physical characteristic, but occasionally differentiation from a lymph node can be difficult. Fine-needle aspiration without ultrasound guidance will be nondiagnostic and the lipocytes will be misinterpreted as contaminants during the penetration process. The ultrasonographic features of a lipoma are virtually

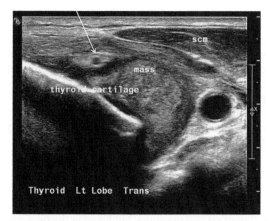

Fig. 3. An inflammatory mass overlying the thyroid cartilage or within the left thyroid lobe can be secondary to a fistula arising from the apex of the pyriform sinus. The arrow points to the actual sinus tract.

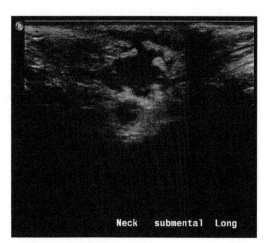

Fig. 1. Subcutaneous abscess.

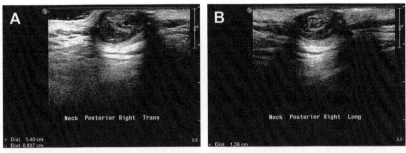

Fig. 4. (*A, B*) Sebaceous cyst in transverse and longitudinal planes. Note that the epicenter of the cyst is at 5 mm from the skin surface.

diagnostic. The overall structure is ovoid and somewhat discrete from the surrounding subcutaneous tissues. Horizontal hyperechoic lines are its hallmark, probably representative of the connective tissue bands that compartmentalize the lipoma. Power Doppler confirms the avascular nature of the mass. Lipomas can be found wherever there is adipose tissue. An example of a parotid lipoma is demonstrated (see **Fig. 5**B). The sonographic features are so typical that the diagnosis can be established on ultrasound study alone.

Salivary Glands

The normal parotid and submaxillary glands have the same ground-glass appearance on ultrasound. Whereas the submaxillary gland is relatively discrete and its dimensions easy to measure, the parotid gland is more difficult to define. Both glands contain large, intermediate, and small ducts and share an intimate relationship with surrounding lymph nodes. In fact, subcapsular lymphadenopathy is usually identified within the parenchyma of the parotid gland. Of all studies

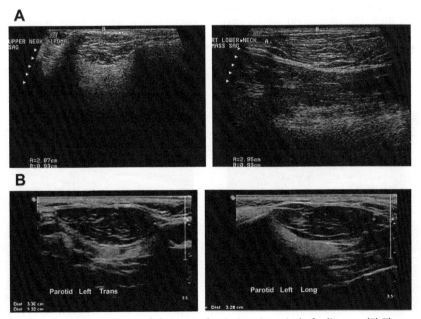

Fig. 5. (*A*) An ovoid subcutaneous mass with horizontal striations is typical of a lipoma. (*B*) The same horizontal striations are indicative of a lipoma in this parotid gland.

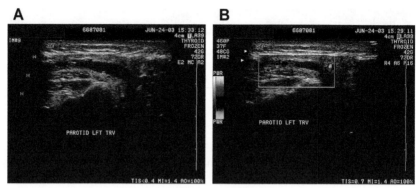

Fig. 6. (*A*) Ectasia of the parotid duct is a typical finding with an obstructing calculus. (*B*) Ectasia of the duct system can be differentiated from a vessel with Doppler assessment.

to investigate parotid pathology, ultrasound is an efficient and cost-effective modality with no radiation exposure. In addition to the initial study, it permits an easy method to efficiently track an inflammatory process over time.

Obstructing Calculus

In this condition, the ductal system will be ecstatic (**Fig. 6**A). The examiner may not be certain whether these conduits are of ductal or vascular origin; the Doppler assessment clarifies the findings with certainty (see **Fig. 6**B). A careful inspection of the ductal system distal to the gland hilum may reveal a discrete hyperechoic density that also demonstrates posterior shadowing artifact (**Fig. 7**). Occasionally, multiple stones may be seen in the duct system, and if they are smaller than the walls of the obstructed duct, the ultrasound waves may cause them to move or vibrate. This can be seen on the real-time images and archived with cine loops (**Fig. 8**).

Diffuse Parotitis

The gland may be inflamed with evidence or obstruction to the main duct system. In this circumstance, there may be edema or areas of heterogeneity throughout the gland and the gland itself is enlarged (**Fig. 9**). It is always a good idea in this circumstance to examine and measure the salivary glands in question bilaterally to compare the normal with abnormal architecture and dimensions.

Sjogren's Syndrome

Lymphoepithelial lesions of the parotid glands have a very distinct image characteristic. The histopathology demonstrates discrete areas throughout the gland that resemble germinal centers in a lymph node (**Fig. 10**). This same appearance can be identified on ultrasound with multiple discrete hypoechoic islands throughout the entire gland. This same echo-appearance is

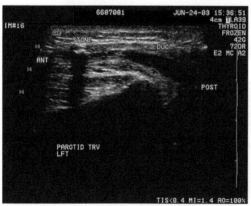

Fig. 7. A distal calculus is identified with posterior shadowing artifact.

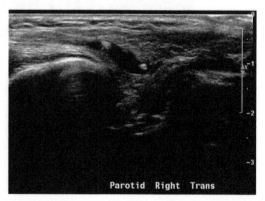

Fig. 8. Multiple calculi within a dilated parotid duct are demonstrated.

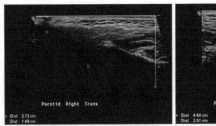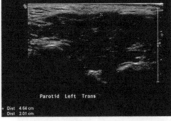

Fig. 9. Diffuse heterogeneous hypoechoic areas within the symptomatic gland are compared with a ground glass appearance of the opposite normal parotid.

noted in Mikulicz disease and recurrent parotitis of childhood.

Parotid Cysts

A single parotid cyst may represent a focal obstruction of a smaller proximal duct, or as a congenital anomaly (first branchial cleft cyst). These cysts are discrete, rounded, anechoic, thinly encapsulated, and demonstrate bright posterior enhancement (**Fig. 11**). Parotid cysts, either single or multiple, may indicate HIV disease. Occasionally, the cyst will contain proteinaceous debris, which presents on ultrasound as discrete punctate areas throughout the cyst (**Fig. 12**). In real time, this debris may demonstrate vibratory movement from the transmitted sound waves.

Tumor

A mass within the parenchyma of either the submaxillary or parotid gland cannot be classified with certainty without cytologic confirmation; however, there are sonographic findings that may

suggest the likelihood of malignancy. The most worrisome abnormalities are irregular ill-defined borders of the mass (**Fig. 13**) with a surrounding normal gland, infiltration of the skin or adjacent muscles, and clear-cut malignant adenopathy of the upper neck in association with a parotid mass. Conversely, a very discrete mass with sharply marginated borders may demonstrate some irregularity in knoblike but confined projections. This type of mass may demonstrate a hypoechoic uniform echo architecture and posterior enhancement artifact, which usually is supportive of a cyst.

The one solid tumor that demonstrates posterior enhancement is a benign mixed tumor (**Fig. 14**). A Warthin tumor may demonstrate characteristics of a cyst, but generally it is not as homogeneous as a mixed tumor and does not demonstrate discrete projections. Parotid malignancies such as adenoid cystic, mucoepidermoid, and acinic cell carcinomas often do not demonstrate specific sonographic features. Thus, fine-needle aspiration cytology is mandatory for any salivary gland mass.

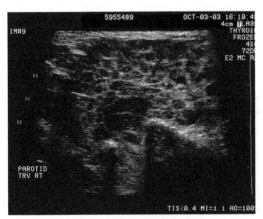

Fig. 10. In Sjogren's syndrome the gland is replaced with a diffuse "honey-combed" appearance.

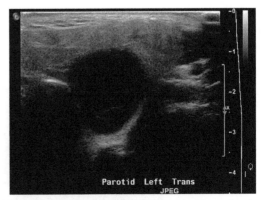

Fig. 11. As with all fluid-filled cysts, those in the parotid have a rounded appearance, are sharply marginated, and demonstrate posterior enhancement.

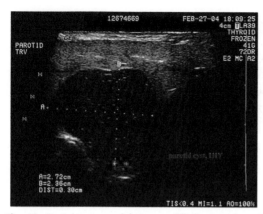

Fig. 12. Proteinaceous debris may fill the interior of the cyst. When multiple, HIV should be suspected.

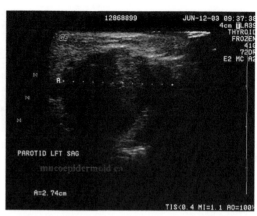

Fig. 13. Parotid masses with irregular margins to the normal gland are strongly suspicious for malignancy.

Occasionally, the precise tissue type cannot be determined; the cytopathologist may be able to diagnose only malignancy, but not much more. Ultrasound-guided core biopsy (16- or 18-gauge) is an excellent adjunctive procedure in this circumstance to allow the pathologist to render a precise diagnosis before surgical intervention. Intraoperative frozen section may similarly plague the pathologist, especially if critical decisions regarding the facial nerve depend on accurate histopathology. A diffuse infiltrative process may be identified as parotid lymphoma, which can be partially characterized with fine-needle aspiration cytology and flow cytometry. Again, core biopsy under ultrasound guidance may be all that is required to precisely identify the lymphoma type and direct appropriate treatment.

Patients with benign mixed tumors who have either tumor spill at surgery or improper management with incisional biopsy are at risk for multiple nodular recurrence. Ultrasound is an excellent modality to carefully map each of the recurrent nodules, either before revision surgery or intraoperatively (**Fig. 15**).

CERVICAL CYSTS

Cystic lesions of the head and neck do not have the same uniform etiology. Some arise from congenital connections with the aerodigestive tract and others develop from obstructing ductal structures or ill-defined degenerative processes within a solid organ or mass.

Thyroglossal Duct Cysts

Although usually midline in location, thyroglossal duct cysts can present as masses off the midline over the thyroid ala, at the thyroid notch and thyrohyoid membrane, and even in the submental triangle. These cysts may be single or multiloculated but always demonstrate the same characteristics: (1) discrete capsule, (2) anechoic echo architecture, and (3) posterior enhancement (**Fig. 16**).

Branchial Cleft Cyst

Second arch cysts are characteristically located at or near the carotid bifurcation and have the

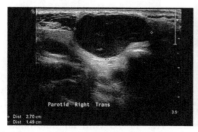
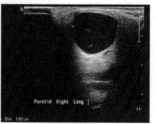

Fig. 14. Pleomorphic adenomas have smooth, sharp margins and may have projections that are still encapsulated. This is the only parotid tumor that demonstrates striking posterior enhancement.

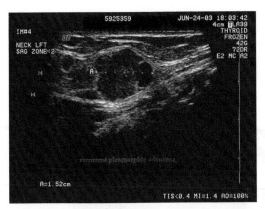

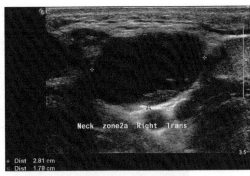

Fig. 17. This cyst in zone II is actually a necrotic lymph node completely replaced by metastatic squamous cell carcinoma.

Fig. 15. Recurrent pleomorphic adenomas may be multiple and these can be carefully mapped with ultrasound before revision surgery or as an intraoperative modality.

same sonographic characteristics as described for the thyroglossal duct cyst. A cyst in the upper neck, often in zone IIa, may represent degeneration of a metastatic squamous cell carcinoma to a lymph node (**Fig. 17**). Occasionally a cyst will be identified on the left side of the neck in zone III or IV and may be associated with recurrent cellulitis or thyroiditis. Frequently, no discrete cyst is identified, only inflammation and occasionally abscess formation. Careful inspection of the

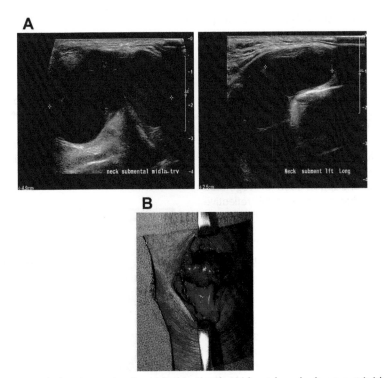

Fig. 16. (*A*) These congenital cysts are closely applied to the thyroid notch and a large cyst is identified over the thyrohyoid region in this sagittal view. (*B*) The operative findings are included for comparison with the actual thyroglossal duct cyst.

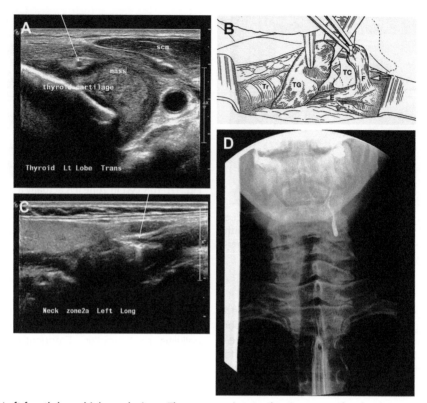

Fig. 18. (*A*) Left fourth branchial pouch sinus. The arrow points to the sinus tract that leads to an inflammatory mass. (*B*) Artist's rendition of fourth branchial pouch sinus. (*C*) Left pharyngeal pouch with entrapped food indicated by refractile sound artifacts. Arrow directs attention to the area of the pouch and refractile food particles. (*D*) Subsequent barium swallow demonstrates the pouch.

area lateral to the thyroid ala and cricoid cartilage may demonstrate a fistulous tract, suggesting the likelihood of a fourth branchial pouch fistula arising from the pyriform sinus (**Fig. 18**A, B). Occasionally, fistulae can arise from the lateral wall of the hypopharynx. One clue to the proper condition may be entrapped food or vegetable matter, which produces an unusual reflective pattern (see **Fig. 18**C). The ultrasound simply allows the clinician to suspect the diagnosis; esophagogram or contrast-enhanced CT swallow defines the pathology with best accuracy (see **Fig. 18**D).

Ranula

A cystic mass in zone I either in the submental region or somewhat lateral may either be superficial to the mylohyoid muscle or demonstrate an extension posteriorly adjacent or deep to the submandibular gland. When the cyst extends posteriorly, it is deep to the mylohyoid muscle (**Fig. 19**). Doppler can be used to confirm the avascular nature of this structure. Needle aspiration confirms the texture and color of the fluid as of salivary origin. An amylase analysis of the fluid may be obtained to confirm a diagnosis of ranula.

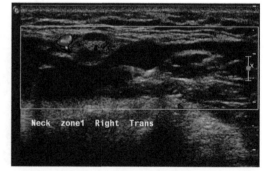

Fig. 19. A plunging ranula extends from the submental region posteriorly to the submandibular gland where the ranula has traversed the mylohyoid.

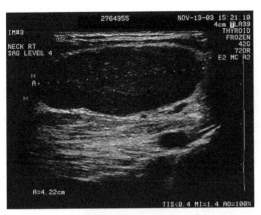

Fig. 20. Large lymphomatous lymph node.

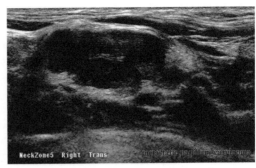

Fig. 22. An irregular border of a lymph node suggests extracapsular extension.

A similar cystic lesion that often has septations and is demonstrated to be macrocystic may reveal straw-colored fluid on aspiration. If cytology demonstrates abundant lymphocytes, the diagnosis of lymphoangioma is confirmed.

LYMPH NODES

Understanding the anatomy of a normal lymph node and its differentiation from one with metastasis or lymphoma is one of the most important advantages of head and neck ultrasound. In addition to the accurate identification of a pathologic node that may not be evident on palpation often has important therapeutic implications. It is critical to identify significant adenopathy but also to accurately describe its precise location into an appropriate neck zone. In addition to these important qualifying features, ultrasound in conjunction with

fine-needle aspiration cytology provides accurate and relatively noninvasive diagnostic capabilities. Finally, simple chemical assessment of the aspirate may allow definitive diagnostic information, ie, thyroglobulin identification in a node confirms the presence of metastatic thyroid carcinoma and a node positive for calcitonin confirms metastatic medullary cancer of the thyroid.

There is no single sonographic characteristic of a lymph node that defines malignancy, but rather a composite of findings may allow the clinician to be strongly suspicious.[1] The following are features that may suggest malignant lymphadenopathy:

1. Large size—The average lymph node is 1 to 1.5 cm in greatest dimension. Upper cervical nodes, especially in the child or adolescent, may be 2 or 3 times this average size but will retain other characteristics of normalcy. Most nodes that are abnormally large, ie, 4 cm in

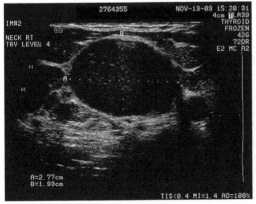

Fig. 21. In a rounded lymph node, transverse and sagittal dimensions are nearly equivalent.

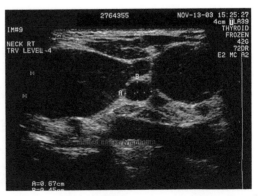

Fig. 23. Multiple nodes are often representative of malignancy, in this instance a non-Hodgkin lymphoma.

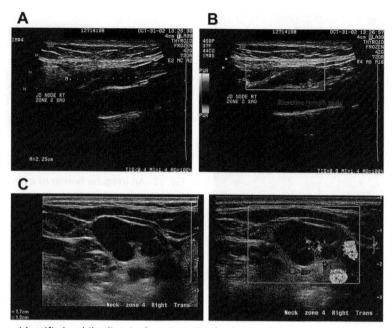

Fig. 24. (*A*) When identified, a hilar line is characteristic of a benign lymph node. (*B*) Power Doppler demonstrates the axial vessel along the hilum in this same node. (*C*) A round or large node may simply be hyperplastic and not malignant. When a well-defined hilar vasculature is identified, malignancy is less likely.

greatest dimension also demonstrate other abnormalities (**Fig. 20**).

2. Rounded shape—The average benign node is at least twice as long as it is wide. Exceptions to this measurement relationship are submental nodes that are often round rather than ovoid in shape. Lymphomatous nodes are often large and rounded (**Fig. 21**). The S/L ratio is an abbreviation sometimes used to illustrate this point. A short/long ratio of less than 0.5 is generally regarded as a normal value.

3. Irregular margin—Nodes that are irregular are also usually larger than average. The capsule of the node may be ill defined and incomplete when malignant cells extend into perinodal soft tissue or adjacent muscle. This is one of the most significant ultrasonographic features of malignancy (**Fig. 22**).

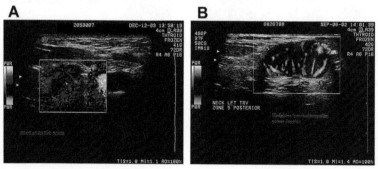

Fig. 25. (*A*) Peripheral vascularity is demonstrated in a node with metastatic squamous cell carcinoma. (*B*) Transnodal vessels are seen in gray scale in this lymphomatous node.

4. Multiple nodes—Nodes that are matted together or multiple in one or more zones are likely to be pathologic. Inflammatory conditions such as tuberculosis or cat scratch disease may demonstrate these features. Lymphomatous nodes are often multiple in number (**Fig. 23**).

5. Loss of hilar architecture—The nodal hilum is usually seen in a normal lymph node. This is a central hyperechoic linear structure that locates the artery, emerging vein, and efferent lymphatics of the node (**Fig. 24A, B**). Absence of this hilar line may suggest that the node is replaced by an infiltrative process. In hyperplastic lymphadenopathy, the hilum is usually preserved and the vasculature may be more evident than normal with power Doppler (see **Fig. 24C**). The normal hilum may be quite thick in structure or even occupy a significant portion of the nodal substance.

6. Peripheral vascularity—Every enlarged or suspect node should be examined with Doppler. Depending on the Doppler resolution of the ultrasound machine as well as dimension of the actual vessels, the hilar vasculature may not be apparent even in a normal node. If the axial hilar vessels are identified, the node is normal and not neoplastic. If there is peripheral hypervascularity surrounding the node or transnodal multiple vessels, angiogenic vessels may be responsible, indicative of metastatic malignancy (**Fig. 25A, B**).

7. Echogenicity—Homogeneous echo architecture in a large rounded node may reflect the "fish flesh" gross appearance seen in lymphomatous nodes (**Fig. 26**). Any cystic anechoic nodes are suspicious for metastatic papillary carcinoma (**Fig. 27**). Areas of anechoic

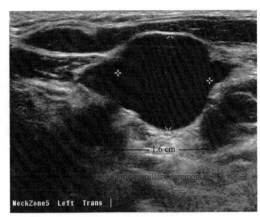

Fig. 27. This cystic node with microcalcifications is typical of metastatic papillary carcinoma.

echogenicity within a node may suggest necrosis and metastatic malignancy (**Fig. 28**).

8. Calcification—Coarse calcifications are seen in a variety of benign conditions and are typically discrete areas of hyperechogenicity with posterior shadowing artifact (**Fig. 29**). These calcifications are common in both benign and malignant thyroid lesions but are uncommon in lymph nodes. Microcalcifications are punctate areas of hyperechoic signal, which in contrast to coarse calcifications do not produce posterior shadowing (**Fig. 30A, B**). When in lymph nodes, they commonly represent metastatic papillary carcinoma (see **Fig. 30C**). They may also be identified in medullary carcinoma (**Fig. 31**). Of all sonographic characteristics, microcalcifications may be the

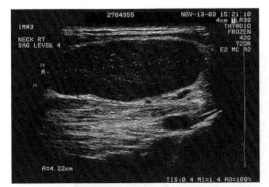

Fig. 26. Homogeneous appearance of a node with non-Hodgkin lymphoma. No axial vascularity can be identified.

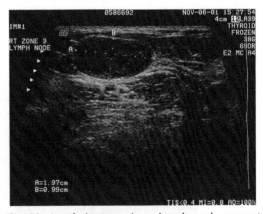

Fig. 28. Anechoic areas in a lymph node suggest necrosis. This node is replaced by areas of metastatic squamous cell carcinoma.

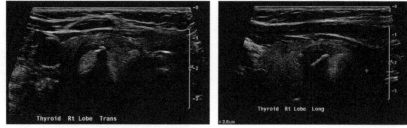

Fig. 29. Coarse thyroid calcifications are densely hyperechoic and demonstrate posterior shadowing artifact.

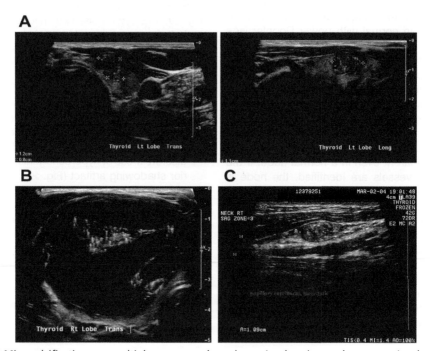

Fig. 30. (*A*) Microcalcifications are multiple punctuate hyperlucencies that do not show posterior shadowing. (*B*) When comet tails extend from punctate hyperlucencies, these are not microcalcifications, although the resemblance is close. They represent crystalline aggregates of colloid and are always indicative of a benign condition. (*C*) Microcalcifications in a lymph node indicate metastatic papillary carcinoma.

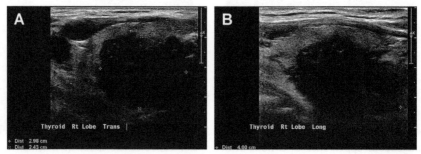

Fig. 31. (*A, B*) Papillary carcinoma of the thyroid demonstrating a few microcalcifications. The anatomic correlates to punctuate microcalcifications are psammoma bodies demonstrated in the histologic image.

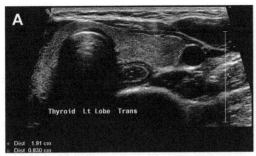
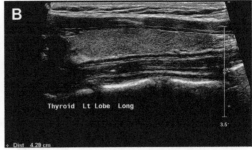

Fig. 32. (*A*) The normal esophagus is a rounded structure in transverse view, usually noted on the left side of the trachea. (*B*) In sagittal view the esophagus is a uniform longitudinal structure alongside the thyroid gland.

most suggestive of metastatic papillary carcinoma to lymph nodes.

The aforementioned nodal characteristics are general guidelines. Most malignant nodes do not demonstrate all of these elements, but when several of these features are identified, suspicion for malignant adenopathy should become a clinical consideration. A recent study by Liao and colleagues[2] nicely illustrates this point. Nodes are assessed for patient age, S/L ratio, internal echogenic characteristics, and vascular pattern and each element is given a weighted score. Cervical nodes are determined to be malignant with scores of equal or greater than 7 with a sensitivity of 100.0%, specificity of 88.0%, and overall

accuracy of 90.1% when compared with actual histology. This scoring system recognizes that no single element defines a malignant node but selects a few key sonographic features that as a composite accurately predict that a cervical node is likely to be malignant.

ESOPHAGUS

The esophagus is a hypoechoic circular structure visualized to the posterolateral aspect of the left lobe of the thyroid on transverse images (**Fig. 32**A). Sagittal views may nicely demonstrate the longitudinal fibers of the esophagus (see **Fig. 32**B). Occasionally, the esophagus is located to the right of the thyroid. A hypoechoic mass

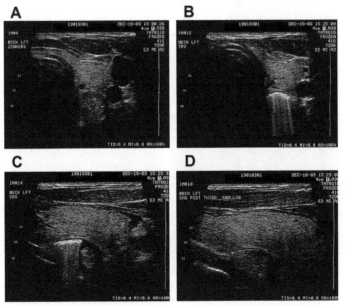

Fig. 33. (*A*) A Zenker diverticulum is suspected when the esophagus seems enlarged and contains material that demonstrates bizarre refractile artifacts. (*B, C, D*) With sequential swallows, the refractile food particles may clear.

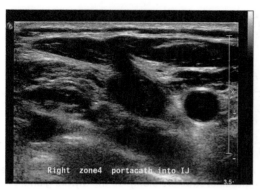

Fig. 34. The internal jugular vein does not illuminate with Doppler when there is thrombosis. In this circumstance, a central-line catheter in the vein for administration of chemotherapy is responsible for the thrombosis.

adjacent to the esophagus, usually noted on the sagittal view, may demonstrate parallel bright transmitted lines in a "sunburst" pattern. These represent artifacts from vegetable or food matter within an esophageal diverticulum, most commonly Zenker type (**Fig. 33**A, B). With repeated swallows this material may actually clear partially or completely (see **Fig. 33**C, D). Pharyngeal pouches

may demonstrate the same refractive food material as demonstrated.

VASCULAR SYSTEM

Dynamic evaluation of a vascular system is one of the most important attributes of cervical high-resolution ultrasound. With a simple touch of a "Doppler button," the examiner can evaluate vascular anatomy, vascular flow pattern of small structures such as lymph nodes, the presence or absence of flow in major structures such as the internal jugular vein, and determine whether a lesion or tumor is of vascular origin. Inflammatory internal jugular vein thrombosis can be identified quite readily (**Fig. 34**) and the suspicion of a tumor thrombus in a patient with thyroid malignancy can have important therapeutic ramifications (**Fig. 35**A, B, C, D). Thyroid nodules are frequently identified incidentally in the course of a carotid vascular study. Conversely, carotid atherosclerosis at the bifurcation may be identified during the course of head and neck ultrasound stimulating appropriate clinical referral (**Fig. 36**).

Cystic lesions of the parotid or zone I may demonstrate multiple septations. This lesion may be either a lymphangioma or hemangioma and Doppler can easily differentiate them. The hemangioma has

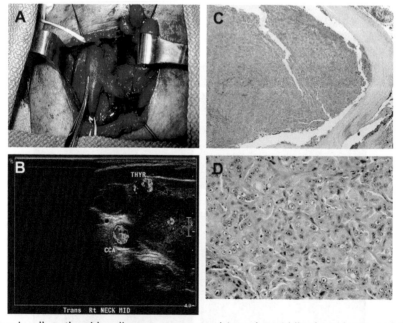

Fig. 35. (*A*) Occasionally a thyroid malignancy may extend into the middle thyroid vein and thereafter the internal jugular vein (IJV). (*B*) Transverse ultrasound image with Doppler demonstrates absence of IJV flow. (*C*) A cross section of the IJV demonstrates the thrombosis (hematoxylin and eosin, low power). (*D*) Histology of the thrombus demonstrates a poorly differentiated thyroid carcinoma.

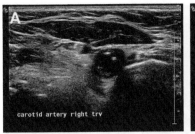
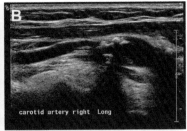

Fig. 36. (*A, B*) Atherosclerosis of the common carotid artery is indicated by calcification at the carotid bulb.

large vascular spaces between the septae and lymphangioma demonstrates a lack of significant vascularity (**Fig. 37**A, B, C, D). Fine-needle aspiration of the lymphangioma reveals straw-colored fluid and abundant lymphocytes on cytology. A mass effect in the parotid may also represent a vascular anomaly. When a large vessel loop is noted on Doppler study, a more definitive vascular study such as CT angiogram may be warranted (**Fig. 38**A, B).

MISCELLANEOUS MASSES

A mass lesion in zone IIa may be a benign or malignant hyperplastic lymph node, second branchial cleft cyst, degenerated metastatic lymph node, or a neurogenic or vascular tumor. A carotid body tumor will demonstrate a mass at the bifurcation, separation of the internal and external carotid arteries, and a hypervascular parenchyma (**Fig. 39**A, B). Doppler will demonstrate that the tumor vascularity arises from an

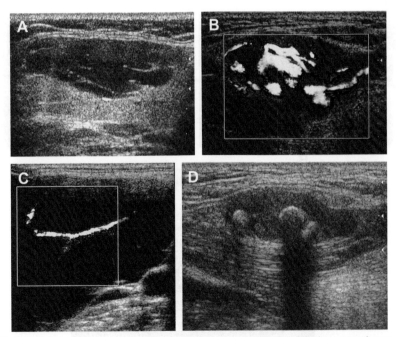

Fig. 37. (*A*) A hemangioma of the parotid gland demonstrates septations. (*B*) The parenchyma of the hemangioma demonstrates hypervascularity. (*C*) When vascularity is confined to the septations and absent in the parenchyma, a lymphangioma is suspected. (*D*) Calcifications are demonstrated in this hemangioma.

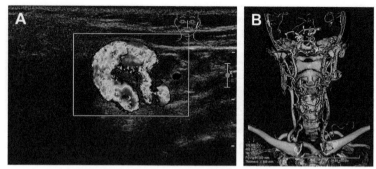

Fig. 38. (*A*) A parotid mass studied with Doppler demonstrates a large vessel loop. The ultrasound led to the diagnostic CT angiogram. (*B*) The vessel loop is from an anomalous internal carotid artery.

independent vessel from the external carotid system, usually the ascending pharyngeal artery (see **Fig. 39**C). Neurogenic tumors arising from the sympathetic chain displace the carotid artery anteriorly and demonstrate a Horner syndrome clinically (**Fig. 40**A, B). A characteristic taper at the inferior end of the mass represents the nerve of origin. A neurofibroma of the cervical plexus may also displace the carotid anteromedially, but there is no Horner syndrome. Again, a taper of the mass at the inferior end will indicate the association with the nerve of origin. Power Doppler confirms that the mass is not a vascular lesion.

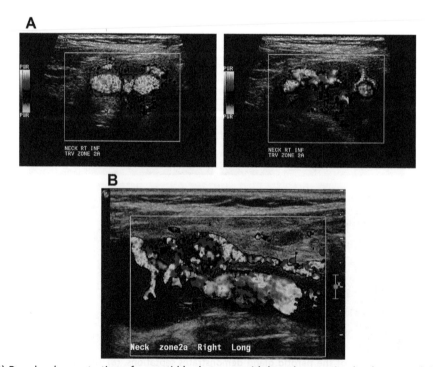

Fig. 39. (*A*) Doppler demonstration of a carotid body tumor with broad separation by the mass of the internal and external carotid arteries. (*B*) Sagittal Doppler view demonstrates the precise vascular supply to the carotid body tumor from the ascending pharyngeal artery.

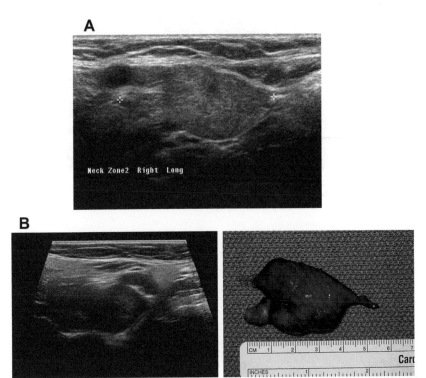

Fig. 40. (*A*) A neurofibroma arising from the sympathetic chain is demonstrated in zone IIa. (*B*) A comparison of the ultrasound image and actual pathology reveals the precision of ultrasound including the taper at the nerve exit from the tumor.

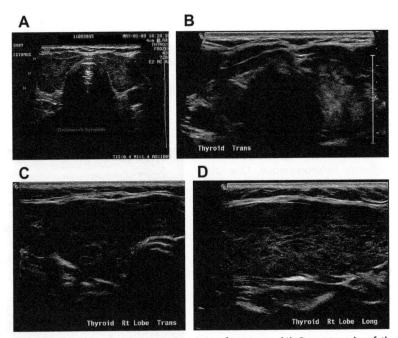

Fig. 41. Hashimoto thyroiditis may demonstrate a variety of patterns. (*A*) One example of thyroiditis demonstrates the typical disappearance of thyroid parenchyma. (*B*) Another form may demonstrate thyromegaly and hypoechoic streaking and pseudonodule formation. (*C, D*) A "Swiss cheese" pattern is frequently noted on ultrasound.

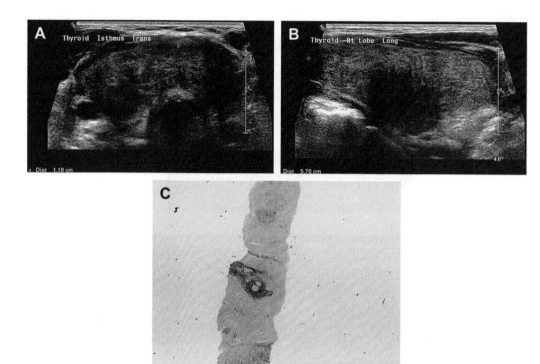

Fig. 42. (*A, B*) A rare inflammatory condition, Riedel struma, demonstrates diffuse fibrosis on both sagittal and transverse views. (*C*) A core biopsy is frequently required as the fibrosis does not demonstrate on fine-needle aspiration (H & E, low power).

THYROID LESIONS

Thyroid ultrasound has been covered in The Role of Ultrasound in Thyroid Disorders elsewhere in this issue. Here, some of the more common entities are described.

Hashimoto Thyroiditis

There are several distinct images that are demonstrative of thyroiditis (**Fig. 41**A, B). One of the key hallmarks of thyroiditis is the diffuse nature of the condition and bilateral and isthmus involvement. The thyroid is diffusely heterogeneous. One of the more typical images is a "Swiss cheese" pattern. There may be multiple pseudo nodule formations or hypoechoic streaking throughout the gland. The thyroid is relatively hypovascular. Riedel struma, a rare inflammatory condition, may resemble thyroiditis (**Fig. 42**A, B).

The rigid texture and lack of cellularity on fine-needle aspiration cytology may require core biopsy for definitive diagnosis (see **Fig. 42**C).

Graves Disease

The thyroid may be significantly enlarged or even relatively normal in size. Power Doppler always demonstrates diffuse hypervascularity (**Fig. 43**).

Multinodular Goiter

There are many sonographic variations of nodular goiter. Nodules may be hypoechoic, hyperechoic, or anechoic and vary in size and position. Coarse calcifications are common. Occasionally, the inferior extent of the thyroid cannot be determined on ultrasound, requiring CT scan to determine the

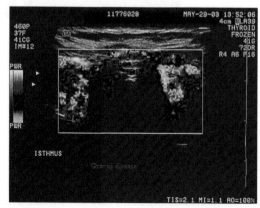

Fig. 43. In contrast to an enlarged thyroid gland with Hashimoto thyroiditis, Graves disease demonstrates diffuse hypervascularity with power Doppler.

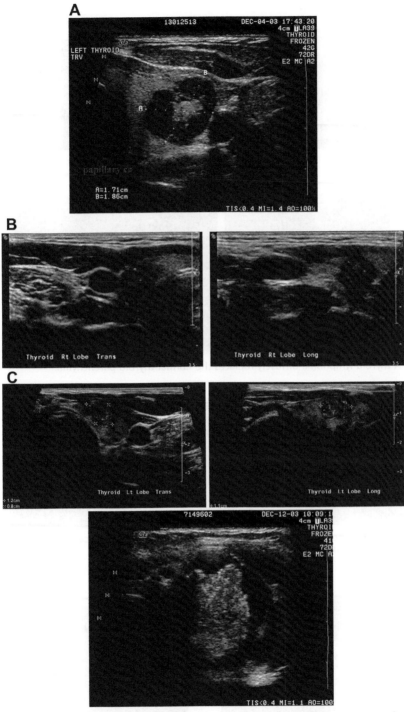

Fig. 44. Papillary carcinoma has several identifying features on ultrasound. (*A*) The mass may be cystic. (*B*) The margins may be irregular. (*C*) Diffuse microcalcifications are common. (*D*) Power Doppler often demonstrates that the mass is hypervascular.

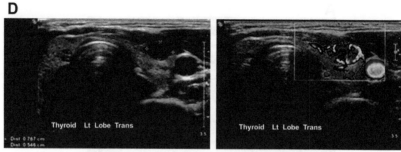

Fig. 44. (continued)

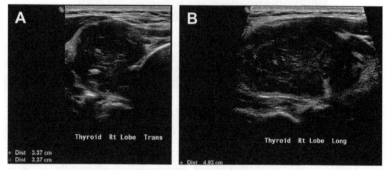

Fig. 45. (A, B) A thyroid lymphoma diffusely replaces the normal thyroid parenchyma.

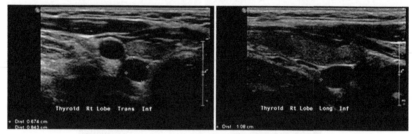

Fig. 46. An inferior parathyroid adenoma is demonstrated in an extracapsular location with hypoechoic architecture and a typical ovoid configuration.

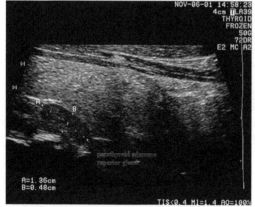

Fig. 47. A superior parathyroid adenoma in its cardinal position.

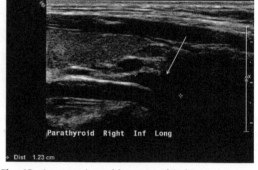

Fig. 48. An ectopic and hypertrophied superior parathyroid gland is demonstrated on this sagittal view of a patient with MEN I. The arrow points to the superior adenoma adjacent to the more typically located enlarged inferior parathyroid gland.

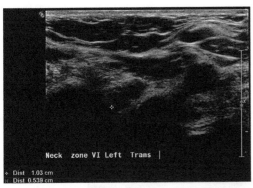

Fig. 49. Inferior parathyroid gland within the thymus.

degree of substernal extension. The isthmus must be carefully assessed, as it is easy to forget that it can harbor large nodules or significant pathology. One of the most difficult concepts in assessment of multinodular goiter is to determine which nodules to biopsy. The "dominant" nodule is the largest of multiple nodules and traditionally the one most likely to be biopsied; however, there are other nodule characteristics that may require biopsy. Irregularity, infiltration of strap muscles, hypervascularity, and microcalcifications are some of the features that demand biopsy.

Single Nodule

A single anechoic nodule that has a distinct hypoechoic halo and is hypovascular often represents a follicular lesion. A single nodule that reveals microcalcifications, irregular margins, and hypervascularity on Doppler is suspicious for papillary carcinoma (**Fig. 44**A, B, C, D). Medullary carcinoma can demonstrate microcalcifications.

Anechoic nodules may be either adenomatous or cysts. Of course, obvious associated suspicious adenopathy should raise the possible question of a relationship to the single thyroid nodule. Thyroid lymphoma is a more diffuse process and replaces the entire lobe or full gland (**Fig. 45**A, B).

PARATHYROID LESIONS

The normal parathyroid glands are below the resolution ability of ultrasound. Primary hyperparathyroidism is most commonly the result of a single adenoma. The parathyroid adenoma is hypoechoic and nearly anechoic in architecture. It is also classically located. The inferior adenoma is at or near the inferior pole of the thyroid and immediately adjacent to the thyroid capsule (**Fig. 46**). The superior parathyroid adenoma is at or craniad to the midpoint of the thyroid gland (**Fig. 47**). When ectopic, the superior parathyroid may even be inferior to the position of the normal inferior parathyroid gland and may locate to the area adjacent to the esophagus (**Fig. 48**). Frequently the inferior parathyroid adenoma is in the thymic tongue and is still identifiable with ultrasound (**Fig. 49**).

Diffuse hyperplasia is suspected when 2 or more enlarged parathyroids are identified (**Fig. 50**A, B). Occasionally, a parathyroid adenoma is difficult to distinguish from a hyperplastic lymph node. One of the key differentiating features is the vascular pattern of the adenoma on Doppler. A discrete vessel (parathyroid artery, a branch of the inferior thyroid artery) is identified anterior to the adenoma and ends bluntly in the parenchyma of the mass (**Fig. 51**A, B, C, D). In contrast, the vascular pattern of a lymph node classically arborizes within the node and a dominant adjacent vessel is less likely (**Fig. 52**). When a parathyroid

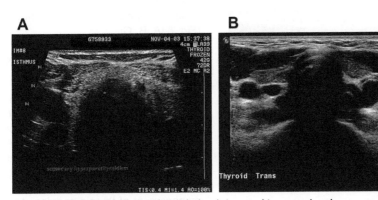

A   **B**

Fig. 50. (A) Marked enlargement of all parathyroid glands is noted in secondary hyperparathyroidism from renal disease. (B) Three enlarged parathyroid glands are demonstrated in this single transverse plane in a patient with MEN I.

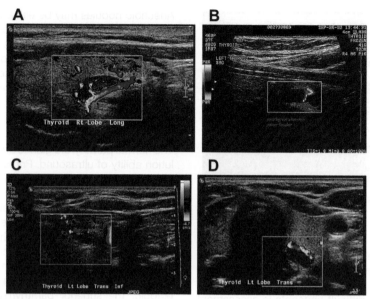

Fig. 51. (*A, B, C, D*) The vascular pattern of a typical parathyroid adenoma demonstrates a well-defined parathyroid artery that ends bluntly in the adenoma parenchyma. Four separate cases are demonstrated.

adenoma cannot be identified in any cardinal position, an ectopic position is likely. The thymus, carotid sheath and area adjacent to the pyriform sinus are consistent regions of investigation. The intrathyroidal adenoma can be identified on preoperative ultrasound (**Fig. 53**A). Again, a dominant single vessel can usually be noted entering the intrathyroidal adenoma, which otherwise cannot be distinguished sonographically from a simple thyroid adenoma. Occasionally a large intrathyroidal adenoma becomes cystic and may be misinterpreted as a complex thyroid nodule or cyst

![Neck Left zone3 Long ultrasound image]

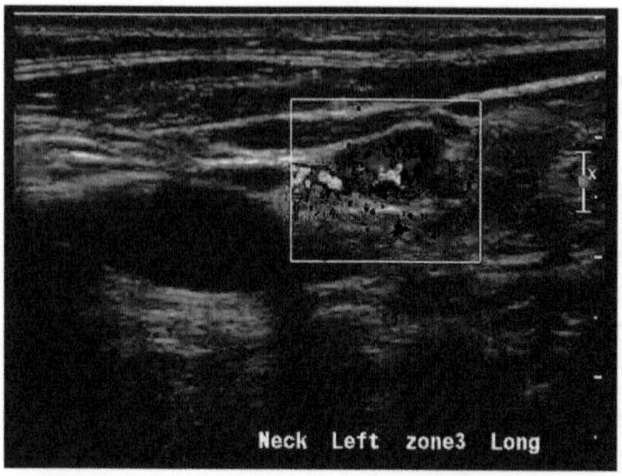

Fig. 52. In contrast to the vascular pattern of a parathyroid adenoma, a hyperplastic lymph node demonstrates an arborizing pattern within the node.

(see **Fig. 53**B). In this circumstance, a fine-needle aspiration for a parathyroid hormone will determine the true nature of the lesion in question.

TEMPOROMANDIBULAR JOINT AND MANDIBLE

Temporomandibular joint arthritis or other deficits may be identified on ultrasound. Occasionally, a joint effusion is noted when one side is compared with the normal asymptomatic joint. A cyst in the parotid gland adjacent to the mandibular condyle may be of synovial origin from the joint. An example of this circumstance demonstrates the precise connection of the cyst to the joint, which was not determined on any other imaging modality including fine-cut CT scan (**Fig. 54**A, B, C).

ULTRASOUND BY THE OTOLARYNGOLOGIST FOR DIAGNOSIS

These are but a few examples of the comprehensive application of ultrasound to the diagnosis and management of head and neck lesions. In the hands of the clinician, real-time examination of relevant anatomy adds immeasurably to the understanding of the condition at hand. This procedure allows more efficient and precise management of thyroid nodules at selected intervals because the same examiner is performing the assessment each time. Any lesion of interest

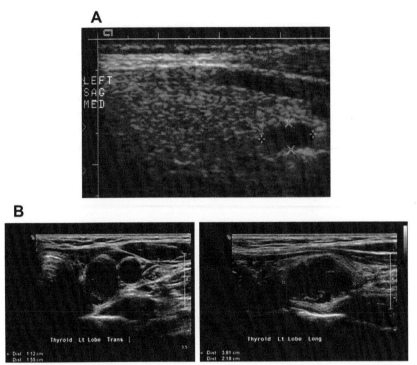

Fig. 53. (*A*) An intrathyroidal parathyroid adenoma is completely surrounded by normal thyroid parenchyma. (*B*) The intrathyroidal parathyroid adenoma may demonstrate cystic degeneration and require parathyroid hormone assessment of its fluid for confirmation.

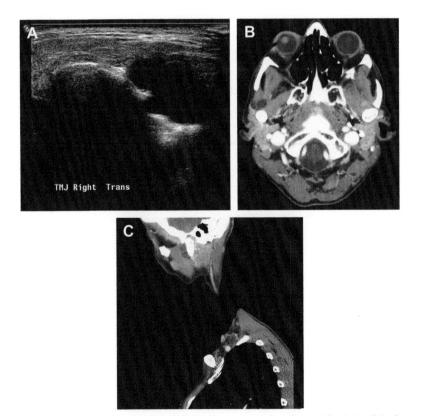

Fig. 54. (*A*) A cystic mass near the temporomandibular joint may not be of parotid origin. This ultrasound demonstrates the connection between this cyst and the joint, which confirms the diagnosis of a synovial cyst. (*B, C*) CT scans do not adequately demonstrate this relationship.

is amenable to fine-needle aspiration cytology, which often can be performed during the same visit. This process is more efficient for patients and will be cost effective. Most importantly, when ultrasound becomes common practice for clinicians, new previously undetermined applications of this modality will evolve and add to the body of diagnostic knowledge.

REFERENCES

1. Ahuja A, Evans R. Practical head and neck ultrasound. London: Greenwich Medical Media Limited; 2000.
2. Liao LJ, Wang CT, Young YH, et al. Real-time and computerized sonographic scoring system for predicting malignant cervical lymphadenopathy. Head and Neck 2010;32:594–8.

The Expanding Utility of Office-Based Ultrasound for the Head and Neck Surgeon

Jeffrey M. Bumpous, MD[a], Gregory W. Randolph, MD[b],*

KEYWORDS

- Ultrasound • Head and neck surgery
- Office-based ultrasound

ULTRASOUND FOR THE HEAD AND NECK SURGEON

Ultrasound has increasingly moved from being a modality confined to the radiology department to an active diagnostic and therapeutic aid available to the head and neck at the point of patient care.[1] Ultrasound as a modality offers several advantages, including small size, low cost of instrumentation, steadily improving resolution, and lack of ionizing radiation and can readily be incorporated into a surgeon's algorithm for determining risk of malignancy in lymph nodes and thyroid nodules.[1,2] The clinical application of ultrasound for head and neck surgeons continues to evolve with increasing levels of information derived from the technology, increasing numbers of practitioners becoming familiar with ultrasound, and a rapidly expanding volume of literature. A PubMed search from January 1, 2000, to January 1, 2010, revealed 1800 articles regarding the use of ultrasound in the head and neck (almost 5 articles per day).

The use of ultrasound has become increasingly sophisticated with 2-D imaging as well as Doppler flow, which help characterize vascular patterns, in particular for hyperechoic foci within the thyroid gland to distinguish vessels from cystic masses.

Addition of advanced ultrasound techniques, such as elastography, increases ultrasound specificity in detecting thyroid malignancy.[2,3] Increasingly, there are ultrasound-related courses and didactic training for practicing physicians. Formal ultrasonography head and neck curricula exist, for example, in the postgraduate medical education head and neck ultrasound course of the American College of Surgeons. In order to optimize safety and accuracy of ultrasonography in an otolaryngology practice, systematic application of the modality with full knowledge of the strengths and weaknesses of the modality must be appreciated.[2]

BASICS OF ULTRASOUND TECHNOLOGY FOR THE OFFICE

There are many clinical ultrasound systems available for clinical use in the office and at the bedside. Small size, portability, and affordability of this equipment have made it more available and attractive to clinical practice. System requirements can be viewed as basic and advanced. More advanced components may require increasing levels of training for accurate use. **Table 1** lists basic and advanced requirements for office-based ultrasound systems.[1]

This article was previously published in the December 2010 issue of *Otolaryngologic Clinics of North America*.
[a] Department of Surgery, University of Louisville, University Surgical Associates, PSC, 401 East Chestnut Street, Suite 710, Louisville, KY 40202, USA
[b] Massachusetts Eye and Ear Infirmary, 243 Charles Street, Boston, MA 02114, USA
* Corresponding author.
E-mail address: Gregory_Randolph@meei.harvard.edu

Ultrasound Clin 7 (2012) 191–195
doi:10.1016/j.cult.2011.12.003

Table 1
Basic and advanced requirements for head and neck office-based ultrasound systems

Component	Basic	Advanced
Ultrasound machine	1. High frequency (7.5–14 MHz) 2. A and B modes 3. Color-coded duplex (enhances differentiation of cystic areas and vascularity)	1. 3-D ultrasound 2. Elastography
Education	1. American College of Surgeons course 2. American Academy of Otolaryngology	1. Radiological Society of North America 2. American Association of Clinical Endocrinologists

Data from Lyshchilk AH. Thyroid gland tumor. Radiology 2005;237(1):202–11.

EVALUATION TECHNIQUE: AN ANATOMIC APPROACH

Development of a systematic approach to performing head and neck office-based ultrasonography is paramount in order to adequately assess pathology and not miss potentially important clinical findings. **Fig. 1** outlines a systematic approach to head and neck ultrasonography and represents only one organizational scheme. The examination should include the central or visceral compartment of the neck in both longitudinal and transverse planes. Within the central compartment, attention is directed at the endocrine organs (thyroid and parathyroid), trachea, esophagus, and paratracheal and prelaryngeal and pretracheal lymph nodes. In the postoperative neck of well-differentiated thyroid cancer patients, accurate reporting of size, location, and character of lymph nodes is important to assess for disease progression. The

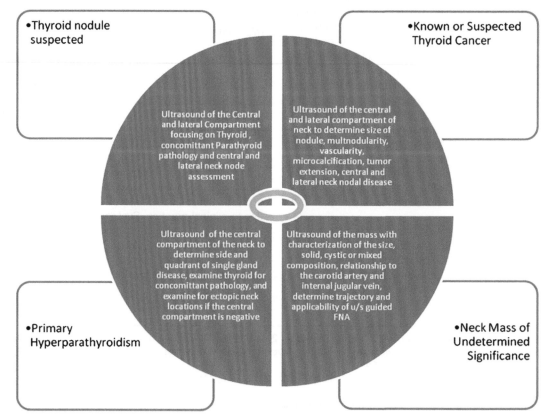

• Thyroid nodule suspected

Ultrasound of the Central and lateral Compartment focusing on Thyroid, concomittant Parathyroid pathology and central and lateral neck node assessment

• Known or Suspected Thyroid Cancer

Ultrasound of the central and lateral compartment of neck to determine size of nodule, multnodularity, vascularity, microcalcification, tumor extension, central and lateral neck nodal disease

Ultrasound of the central compartment of the neck to determine side and quadrant of single gland disease, examine thyroid for concomittant pathology, and examine for ectopic neck locations if the central compartment is negative

Ultrasound of the mass with characterization of the size, solid, cystic or mixed composition, relationship to the carotid artery and internal jugular vein, determine trajectory and applicability of u/s guided FNA

• Primary Hyperparathyroidism

• Neck Mass of Undetermined Significance

Fig. 1. Systematic application of head and neck ultrasonography.

lateral neck must also be evaluated in patients with thyroid cancer; failure to do so results in poor sensitivity of the examination in detection of lymphadenopathy.[1,2,4]

THYROID ULTRASOUND

With respect to the thyroid gland, the dimensions of both lobes and the isthmus should be assessed and recorded, which requires assessment in the longitudinal and transverse planes. Size, location, and echo characteristics should also be recorded. Vascular patterns surrounding nodules from Doppler flow may provide etiologic clues.[1,2,4] Any calcifications should be noted and preferably recorded as static images. A pattern of microcalcification in a nodule significantly increases the risk that the nodule may be malignant. In the multinodular thyroid gland, ultrasound is particularly helpful in recognizing areas within the gland that are at higher risk of malignancy, such as nodules greater than 1 cm and those possessing hypervascularity and microcalcification.[2] Limitations of ultrasound in thyroid assessment include assessment of substernal extent of the gland, predicting airway invasion, distinguishing coexistent lymph node from parathyroid pathology, and lack of definitive pathologic characteristics in the context of a multinodular gland.[1,4] **Table 2** lists common characteristics of thyroid malignancy on ultrasound.

PARATHYROID ULTRASOUND

The parathyroid glands in the normal state are difficult to precisely identify in many state-of-the-art imaging modalities, including ultrasound.[5] In the case of primary hyperparathyroidism, however, ultrasound of the central compartment may be diagnostic of single-gland disease (adenoma).

Table 2
Ultrasound characteristics of thyroid malignancy
Size >1 cm and solid
Microcalcification
Central blood flow pattern
Strain index >4 on offline elastograms (96% specificity, 82% sensitivity)
Margin regularity score (88% specificity, 36% sensitivity)
Tumor area ratio >1 (92% specificity, 46% sensitivity)

Data from Welkoborsky HJ. Ultrasound usage in the head and neck surgeon's office. Curr Opin Otolaryngol Head Neck Surg 2009;17(2):116–21; and Lyshchilk AH. Thyroid gland tumor. Radiology 2005;237(1):202–11.

Anatomic relationships to the trachea, larynx, esophagus, thyroid, and carotid sheath contents may allow for identification of diseased parathyroid glands and provide information regarding side and upper or lower position.

In cases of positive nuclear medicine studies, such as technetium 99m sestamibi scan, ultrasound may provide more refined information regarding anatomic location of the adenoma than nuclear medicine study alone.[5,6] In cases of suspicious yet equivocal nuclear medicine evaluations, office-based ultrasonography can provide concordance. If the two examinations are concordant, the correlations with successful unilateral surgical exploration and correction of hypercalcemia are greater than 95%.[7] Several studies have demonstrated success in localizing single-gland disease in cases of negative nuclear medicine studies, arguably making this modality the most useful modality in parathyroid localization; this in part may be a result of high-resolution ultrasound; when read by an experienced ultrasonographer, it may allow identification parathyroid adenomas as small as 0.5 cm.[5]

In clinical practice, localization of single- versus multiple-gland disease may often be aided by office ultrasound and nuclear medicine assessment. Additionally, ectopic locations in the lateral neck and submandibular triangle are readily accessible for ultrasound examination, but mediastinal ectopic glands are not often identified with ultrasound. Critics of ultrasound localization of parathyroid adenoma suggest that there are limitations in resolution (without high-resolution scanners), potential confusion with paratracheal lymph nodes, and difficulty in imaging below the clavicles.[5–7]

NECK LYMPHATICS ULTRASOUND

Examination of the lymphatics of the neck by office-based ultrasound is pertinent in evaluation of myriad pathologies, including upper aerodigestive, thyroid, and parathyroid malignancy as well as benign lymphadenopathy and other neck masses. Size greater than 1 cm, clustering of nodes, rounding of shape, peripheral vascularity, cystic (hyperechoic) change, microcalcification, and loss of a distinguishable fatty hilum on ultrasound are all characteristics of malignancy within cervical nodes.[8] Ultrasound provides an objective means of documenting lymph node size, location, and characteristics and can, therefore, be useful in following equivocal areas for progression in size. In particular, ultrasound is useful for post-thyroidectomy follow-up of patients with an established diagnosis of well-differentiated thyroid carcinoma. Early baseline examination (with or without needle biopsy) and subsequent follow-up examinations provide a context for evaluating both central compartment and lateral lymph nodes for growth.[2,8–10] Preoperative ultrasound evaluation of the lateral neck in high-risk patients with well-differentiated thyroid cancer may allow for more appropriate inclusion or exclusion of lateral compartment lymphadenectomy.[10] In cases of elevated thyroglobulin in post-thyroidectomy, well-differentiated thyroid carcinomas, ultrasound can provide a low-cost and accurate means of reassessing the thyroid bed and cervical nodal basin. Ultrasound represents an effective and low-cost modality that may supplement or even obviate iodine scan or PET scan in situations where thyroglobulin is elevated.[11] Additionally, ultrasound provides superior opportunity for needle-based biopsy than nuclear medicine studies; is less expensive than other image-guided biopsy modalities, such as CT and MRI; and may also be useful in directed needle-based interventions in poorly accessible or nonpalpable areas (ie, alcohol injection of small metastatic nodes).[2,8,9,11]

OFFICE-BASED HEAD AND NECK ULTRASOUND BIOPSY

Ultrasound-guided needle aspiration biopsy is a well-accepted modality for biopsy of head and neck masses from salivary to endocrine to lymphatic tissues.[2] Ultrasound-guided needle biopsy of head and neck masses should be preceded by adequate history, physical examination, and diagnostic ultrasound of the pathology in question as well as surrounding head and neck structural relationships.[1,2,4,9] Optimal diagnostic success occurs when there is communication between the clinician and pathologist to make certain there is adequate sample retrieved and that the sample is processed appropriately. Office-based ultrasound-guided biopsy of thyroid, parathyroid, lymphatic and other neck masses allows for more prompt diagnosis. The technical process of ultrasound-guided needle biopsy in the head and neck is beyond the scope of this article, but the techniques are increasingly emphasized in well-vetted courses that are available to head and neck surgeons.

THERAPEUTIC APPLICATIONS OF HEAD AND NECK ULTRASOUND

Ultrasound in many areas has become an accepted modality for guidance of therapeutic interventions ranging from alcohol injections to radiofrequency ablation.[11] The literature and experience with ultrasound-guided therapeutic interventions in the head and neck are more limited and without data from large multi-institutional clinical trials. Ultrasound-guided alcohol injection has been reported in ablation of primary thyroid lesions as well as lymph nodes bearing evidence of papillary thyroid carcinoma. Proposed use in parathyroid adenomas is controversial.[11] The lack of a thick capsule in parathyroid adenomas may allow for diffusion of alcohol injections and result in collateral tissue damage, in particular the inferior (recurrent) or superior laryngeal nerves. Cases of recurrent laryngeal nerve paralysis after alcohol injection have been reported.[12,13] Radiofrequency ablation is a modality that is commonly used for areas, such as hepatic lesions. Ultrasound-guided radiofrequency ablation requires additional expertise in understanding microwave technology and its tissue effects. Radiofrequency ablation has been used successfully in the treatment of head and neck lesions and has been reported as an alternative to surgery in selected patients.[14] Pain, hematoma, and voice change are among the reported complications of ultrasound radiofrequency ablation of thyroid lesions.[15,16] Coupled with ultrasound, appropriate training in the interpretation of imaging endpoints, radiofrequency ablation may provide an area of further potential therapeutic intervention for head and neck surgeons.

INTEGRATION OF OFFICE-BASED ULTRASONOGRAPHY

Office-based ultrasonography is increasingly being integrated into the practice of otolaryngology–head and neck surgery. Use of a systematic anatomic-based approach provides increased diagnostic information and opportunities for more refined disease management in thyroid, parathyroid, and upper aerodigestive tract masses and malignancies. Adequate training for appropriate technical execution and clinical interpretation of head and neck disease findings on ultrasound are increasingly available in postgraduate medical education and continuing medical education formats. Unique imaging characteristics, low cost, correlation with clinical examination, and pre-existing anatomic and clinical knowledge of head and neck disease processes make the inclusion of office-based ultrasound for head and neck surgeons an attractive prospect. Ultrasound complements a physical examination in the postoperative or postirradiated neck. In addition to the general diagnostic information of ultrasound, guided biopsy provides an opportunity for precision in the office for fine-needle aspiration of masses that are not readily palpable. Although not well established (due to lack of large-scale clinical trial data), ultrasound-guided therapeutic intervention is an additional area that head and neck surgeons should continue to have awareness of as it enters practice. Ultrasound-based interventions will need critical evaluation for safety and efficacy.

REFERENCES

1. Charous SJ. An overview of office-based ultrasonography: new versions. Otolaryngol Head Neck Surg 2004;131(6):1001–3.
2. Welkoborsky HJ. Ultrasound usage in the head and neck surgeon's office. Curr Opin Otolaryngol Head Neck Surg 2009;17(2):116–21.
3. Lyshchilk AH. Thyroid gland tumor. Radiology 2005; 237(1):202–11.
4. Slough CM. Workup of well-differentiated thyroid carcinoma. Cancer Control 2006;13(2):99–105.
5. Gurney TA. Otolaryngologist-head and neck surgeon performed ultrasonography for identification for parathyroid adenoma localization. Laryngoscope 2008; 118:243–6.
6. Bumpous JM. Surgical and calcium outcomes in 427 patients treated prospectively in an image guided and intraoperative PTH supplemented protocol for primary hyperparathyroidism. Laryngoscope 2009;119:300–6.
7. Lal G. Primary hyperparathyroidism: controversies in surgical management. Trends Endocrinol Metab 2003;14(9):417–22.
8. Gritzman NH. Sonography of soft tissue masses of the neck. J Clin Ultrasound 2002;30:356–73.
9. Ahuja A. Sonographic evaluation of cervical lymph nodes. AJR Am J Roentgenol 2004;184:1691–9.
10. Davidson HC. Papillary thyroid cancer: controversies in the management of neck metastasis. Laryngoscope 2008;118:2161–5.
11. Johnson NA. Postoperative surveillance of differentiated thyroid carcinoma: rational, techniques and controversies. Radiology 2008;249(2):429–44.
12. Maus PS. Complications of ultrasound guided percutaneous ethanol injection therapy of the thyroid and parathyroid glands. Ultraschall Med 2005; 26(2):142–5.
13. Brzac H. Ultrasonography-guided therapeutic procedures in the neck. Acta Med Croatica 2009;63(3): 21–7.
14. Baek J. Benign predominantly solid thyroid nodules: prospective study of efficacy of sonographically guided radiofrequency ablation versus control condition. AJR Am J Roentgenol 2010;194: 1137–42.
15. Jeong WB. Radiofrequency ablation of benign thyroid nodules: safety and imaging follow-up in 236 patients. Eur Radiol 2008;18(6):1244–50.
16. Monchik JM. Radiofrequency ablation and percutaneous ethanol injection treatment for recurrent local and distant well-differentiated thyroid carcinoma. Ann Surg 2006;244(2):296–304.

Role of Ultrasound in Thyroid Disorders

Gerald T. Kangelaris, MD[a], Theresa B. Kim, MD[a,b],
Lisa A. Orloff, MD[c],*

KEYWORDS

- Thyroid ultrasound • Thyroid cancer • Thyroid nodule
- Thyroid FNA • Ultrasonography

(▶) The author has provided several related videos at www.ultrasound.theclinics.com.

HISTORICAL PERSPECTIVE OF THYROID ULTRASOUND

Thyroid ultrasonography commands a central role in the evaluation, diagnosis, and treatment of thyroid disorders. Ultrasound has been the standard for imaging of the thyroid gland for many years and is the first-line recommended imaging modality for thyroid nodules.[1,2] Its use in thyroid disorders is widely accepted and the benefits and indications for its use continue to expand. Thyroid ultrasonography has traditionally been under the purview of radiology departments, but in the past decade has been adopted by surgeons and endocrinologists in the office-based setting for evaluation and management of patients with thyroid and other head and neck disorders. Its versatility, speed, safety profile, ability to offer dynamic real-time images, and low cost compared with other radiologic modalities have all contributed to its popularity.

The initial uses of thyroid ultrasonography came at a time when palpable thyroid nodules were surgically excised to establish a pathologic diagnosis. In the late 1960s, ultrasound was used to differentiate between solid and cystic nodules and to measure and track nodule size.[3] Using conventional ultrasonography without the benefit of gray-scale images, clinicians were able to differentiate cysts from cystic degeneration in an adenoma, solid tumors from multinodular goiter, and to detect the presence of thyroiditis with greater than 90% accuracy.[4,5] However, the differentiation of benign versus malignant lesions remained problematic, and in the following decade, investigators began studying whether newer ultrasound technology could help improve surgical and medical decision making by identifying malignant features of thyroid lesions.[6]

In the past 40 years, the role of thyroid ultrasonography has continued to expand and it is currently recommended in the evaluation of all palpable nodules by the American Thyroid Association (ATA), the American Association of Clinical Endocrinologists (AACE), and the Associazione Medici Endocrinologi (AME).[1,2] The thyroid gland is well suited to ultrasound evaluation in part because of the superficial position and easy accessibility of the gland, its distinctive echotexture, and the ability to gain greater anatomic detail than with computed tomography, magnetic resonance imaging, or radionuclide studies. **Table 1** lists some of the goals of and indications for thyroid ultrasonography.

This article reviews the relevant uses of and indications for ultrasound in various thyroid diseases, with particular attention to thyroid nodules and

This article was previously published in the December 2010 issue of *Otolaryngologic Clinics of North America*.
Funding support: the authors have no financial support to disclose.
[a] Department of Otolaryngology – Head & Neck Surgery, University of California, San Francisco, 2380 Sutter Street, 1st Floor, Campus Box 0342, San Francisco, CA 94115, USA
[b] Department of Otolaryngology, Pediatric Otolaryngology, 1 Children's Place, Suite 3S35, St Louis, MO 63110, USA
[c] Department of Otolaryngology–Head & Neck Surgery, University of California, San Francisco, 2380 Sutter Street, 2nd Floor, San Francisco, CA 94115, USA
* Corresponding author.
E-mail address: lorloff@ohns.ucsf.edu

Ultrasound Clin 7 (2012) 197–210
doi:10.1016/j.cult.2011.12.004
1556-858X/12/$ – see front matter © 2012 Elsevier Inc. All rights reserved.

Table 1
Thyroid ultrasonography goals and indications

To better assess palpable thyroid nodules	To facilitate FNA biopsy of a nodule
To determine whether nodularity is present in the patient with an equivocal or difficult physical examination	To assess the remainder of the thyroid gland in the patient with a palpable thyroid nodule
To determine whether characteristics associated with malignancy are present	To screen for thyroid lesions in patients who have been exposed to radiation
To screen for thyroid lesions in patients with other diseases in the neck, such as hyperparathyroidism, who are undergoing treatment planning	To objectively monitor nodules, goiters, or lymph nodes in patients undergoing treatment or observation of thyroid disease
To assess the thyroid and the extrathyroid neck in the patient with thyroid cancer before treatment	To monitor treated patients with thyroid cancer for early evidence of recurrence in the thyroid bed and cervical lymph nodes
To identify thyroid features associated with diseases including thyroiditis and Graves disease	To facilitate therapeutic procedures such as sclerotherapy or laser ablation of thyroid nodules
To help teach regional anatomy and the art of thyroid palpation	To detect undescended thyroid or thyroid agenesis
To monitor fetal thyroid development in utero	To assess the size and location of the neonatal thyroid
To detect goiter as a sign of iodine deficiency	To refine management of patients on therapy such as antithyroid medications
To screen family members of patients with familial forms of thyroid cancer	

Data from Morris LF, Ragavendra N, Yeh MW. Evidence-based assessment of the role of ultrasonography in the management of benign thyroid nodules. World J Surg 2008;32:1253–63; Orloff LA. Head and neck ultrasonography. Plural Publishing; 2008.

cancer. The characteristic ultrasound features of these diseases are described. The associated literature and societal guidelines are discussed.

ROLE OF ULTRASOUND IN THE INITIAL EVALUATION OF THE THYROID NODULE

The ATA and AACE/AME recommend thyroid ultrasound for all patients with suspected thyroid nodules,[1,2] including patients with palpable abnormalities, nodular goiter, and thyroid lesions found incidentally on other imaging modalities. Routine screening thyroid ultrasound is not recommended for the general population because of the high incidence of thyroid nodules. An autopsy study of 821 consecutive patients with clinically normal thyroid glands showed that 50% of patients had at least one thyroid nodule and 36% had nodules greater than 2 cm in size.[7] Palpable thyroid nodules occur in up to 7% of the general adult population, and the incidence of nonpalpable thyroid nodules visible by ultrasound is up to 10 times greater (ie, 70%).[8–10]

Ultrasound evaluation of thyroid nodules in at-risk patients can help confirm the presence of a nodule; objectively characterize the size, location, and appearance of the nodule; evaluate for benign or suspicious features; and evaluate for the presence of other thyroid nodules or cervical lymphadenopathy.[1] Although certain ultrasound characteristics of thyroid nodules are associated with malignancy, fine-needle aspiration (FNA) remains the gold standard for diagnosis. FNA has until recently been recommended for cytologic evaluation of all thyroid nodules greater than 1 cm in diameter or nodules less than 1 cm that exhibit suspicious features.[1,2] The 2009 Revised ATA Guidelines for Management of Thyroid Nodules and Differentiated Thyroid Cancer also include recommendations for FNA of certain thyroid lesions based on ultrasound criteria. These criteria include mixed solid and cystic nodules 1.5 to 2 cm or greater in diameter with any suspicious ultrasound characteristics and predominantly spongiform nodules 2 cm or greater in diameter.[1] Although considered the gold standard, the diagnostic role of FNA is limited by an overall 3% to 5% false-negative rate and a 10% nondiagnostic rate.[11]

The use of ultrasound guidance improves the sensitivity, specificity, and accuracy of FNA compared with palpation-guided FNA in certain populations.[12–15] Ultrasound-guided FNA seems to be most valuable in patients with nonpalpable nodules, small palpable nodules, multiple nodules, partially cystic nodules, or concomitant glandular disease. It is also beneficial for sampling specific areas of a nodule, such as from the solid part of a mixed solid-cystic nodule. Compared with palpation-guided FNA, the use of ultrasound guidance decreased the rate of inadequate samples in palpable nodules 2 cm or smaller from 39% to 23%.[14] Cesur and colleagues[12] found the rates of inadequate FNA samples to be significantly improved in palpable nodules 1.0 to 1.5 cm using ultrasound- versus palpation-guided FNA (37.6% vs 24.4%, $P = .009$), but not for palpable nodules 1.6 cm or larger. Currently, the ATA recommends ultrasound-guided FNA for nodules that are non-palpable, predominately cystic, or located posteriorly in the thyroid lobe, and when repeating FNA for a nodule with an initial nondiagnostic cytology result (Video 1: Ultrasound-guided FNA of a right thyroid nodule. To view video please go to www.ultrasound.theclinics.com).[1]

ULTRASOUND CHARACTERISTICS OF THYROID NODULES

Many investigators have identified ultrasound characteristics of malignant thyroid nodules (**Table 2**). Although these ultrasound characteristics offer high sensitivity, no single criterion offers sufficient specificity to differentiate benign from malignant lesions.[16] However, when taken together, specificity improves. One prospective, observational study compared ultrasound and FNA results with surgical disease conditions in 349 patients and found that performing FNA on nodules with one of 3 ultrasound criteria (microcalcifications, blurred

Table 2 Ultrasound features associated with malignancy	
Margins	Blurred, ill-defined
Halo/rim	Absent
Shape	Irregular, spherical, tall
Echo structure	Solid
Echogenicity	Hypoechoic
Calcifications	Microcalcifications, internal
Vascular pattern	Intranodular, hypervascular
Elastography	Decreased elasticity

Data from Morris LF, Ragavendra N, Yeh MW. Evidence-based assessment of the role of ultrasonography in the management of benign thyroid nodules. World J Surg 2008;32:1253–63.

margins, or hypoechoic pattern) missed only 2% of cancers.[17] Kim and colleagues[18] prospectively analyzed 155 incidentally discovered, nonpalpable, solid thyroid nodules and found a mean number of 2.6 suspicious findings per malignant nodule and an overall sensitivity and specificity of 94% and 66%, respectively.

The next sections discuss ultrasound features of thyroid nodules and their ability to suggest benign versus malignant lesions.

NODULE SIZE

Nodule size has not been found to be significantly predictive of malignancy. The risk of malignancy for palpable thyroid nodules is approximately 10% and several studies suggest a similar incidence of malignancy in nodules smaller than 1 cm.[19–21] Thyroid cancers less than 1 cm in size have been shown to behave clinically similar to larger cancers, and therefore these lesions should be followed with periodic ultrasound surveillance with the option for further evaluation with FNA if growth or suspicious features are observed.[22] The ATA recommends FNA biopsy of subcentimeter nodules if there is a high risk of malignancy (family history of thyroid cancer, history of external beam or ionizing radiation, history of thyroid cancer, or fluorodeoxyglucose-avid thyroid nodules on positron emission tomography) or if there is suspicious concomitant lymphadenopathy, in which case FNA of the lymph node should be performed.[1]

LESION MARGINS AND HALO/RIM

Benign lesions are often associated with a hypoechoic circumferential halo (**Fig. 1**), believed to represent a capsule and compressed thyroid tissue.[23] Neoplasms may display a partial or absent halo,[24] and its presence or absence has been found to be suggestive but not diagnostic.[24,25] Blurred or ill-defined margins have been associated with increased risk of malignancy.[17,24,25] The mobility of the nodule with respect to surrounding structures should be assessed, as fixation suggests malignant invasion of the surrounding tissue.

NODULE SHAPE

Nodule shape has been implicated as having prognostic significance. One retrospective analysis found nodules with a more spherical shape had a higher incidence of malignancy.[23] In contrast, another study found that nodules that are more tall than wide are more likely to harbor cancer.[18] Irregular shape has also been implicated in malignancy.[24]

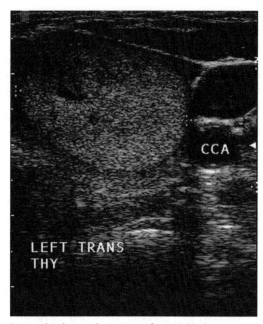

Fig. 1. Thin hypoechoic circumferential halo surrounding a benign thyroid nodule.

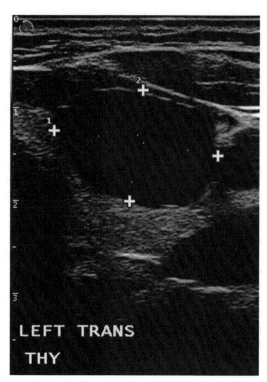

Fig. 2. Cystic degeneration of a benign thyroid nodule.

ECHO STRUCTURE

Many thyroid nodules are cystic or have cystic components, such as cystic degeneration of a follicular adenoma (**Fig. 2**) or in the setting of multinodular goiter. Malignancy has been more closely associated with solid nodules compared with cystic or mixed nodules, with one study finding 121 of 148 (81.8%) histopathologically malignant nodules to be solid.[17,24] Purely cystic nodules are unlikely to be malignant,[26] as are those with a spongiform appearance (**Fig. 3**), defined as an aggregation of multiple microcystic components in more than 50% of the nodal volume.[27,28]

ECHOGENICITY

The echogenicity of a thyroid nodule should be compared with that of surrounding thyroid tissue. Most benign adenomas or adenomatous nodules are slightly hypoechoic when compared with normal thyroid tissue (**Fig. 4**), whereas malignant nodules are frequently markedly hypoechoic (**Fig. 5**).[18,24] In a prospective, observational study of 349 surgically excised thyroid nodules, Cappelli and colleagues[17] found a 3.8 odds ratio of malignancy in solid hypoechoic nodules.

CALCIFICATIONS

The presence of calcifications has variable significance. Peripheral calcification, also referred to as eggshell calcification, is typically considered a benign feature, representing previous hemorrhage and degenerative change (**Fig. 6**). However, coarse calcifications can be seen in malignant nodules, as can microcalcifications, which are strongly associated with an increased risk of malignancy.[17] A total of 45% to 60% of malignant nodules show microcalcifications, as opposed to 7% to 14% of benign nodules.[18,29] Approximately

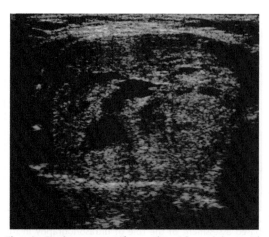

Fig. 3. Benign, spongiform thyroid nodule, with multiple microcystic components.

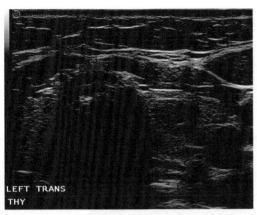

Fig. 4. Slightly hypoechoic benign adenomatous nodule.

60% of patients with microcalcifications were found to have malignant disease.[30] The presence of microcalcifications in malignant nodules is often attributed to psammoma bodies in papillary thyroid carcinoma (PTC) (**Fig. 7** and Video 2: Sagittal view of a primary papillary thyroid carcinoma, showing microcalcifications (sweeping lateral to medial). To view video please go to www.ultrasound.theclinics.com) and is frequently seen in medullary thyroid carcinoma (MTC). Although suggestive of malignancy, the overall specificity of microcalcifications for thyroid carcinoma has been reported to range from 71% to 94%, with a sensitivity of 35% to 72%,[17,31,32] and therefore should not be solely relied on to differentiate benign from malignant lesions.

VASCULAR PATTERN

The vascular pattern around or within a nodule may correlate with the probability of malignancy.

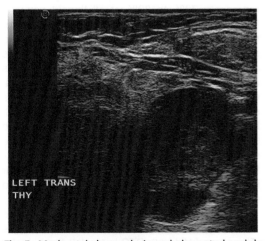

Fig. 5. Moderately hypoechoic and elongated nodule that proved to be a follicular carcinoma.

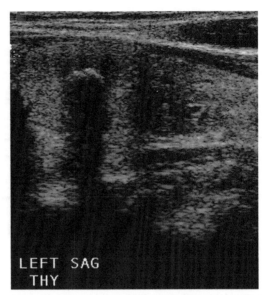

Fig. 6. Peripheral or eggshell calcification in a benign thyroid nodule. Note posterior acoustic shadowing deep to hyperechoic calcification.

Chammas and colleagues[33] classified thyroid nodules according to the pattern of vascularity seen with power Doppler into 5 types: absent blood flow, perinodular flow only, perinodular flow as great or greater than central blood flow, mainly central nodular flow, and central flow only. Nodules with exclusively central blood flow or central blood flow greater than perinodular flow had a higher incidence of malignancy (**Fig. 8**). Follicular carcinomas also tend to show a moderate increase in central vascularity by power Doppler compared with follicular adenomas, which favor peripheral flow (**Fig. 9**).[34] In general, increased vascularity in a thyroid nodule is suggestive of malignancy but should not be considered a pathognomonic feature.

ELASTOGRAPHY

Elastography is the ultrasound measurement of tissue elasticity, a mechanical property reflecting the deformation or distortion of the tissue in response to the application of external compression.[35] In this method, pressure is applied with the ultrasound transducer and used to measure tissue stiffness. The displacement of the strained tissue is estimated by tracking the echo delays in segmented waveforms recorded before and after quasistatic compression. In vitro studies with various tumors show 10-fold greater stiffness of malignant neoplasms compared with normal tissues.[31] Several studies have investigated the application of ultrasound elastography to thyroid

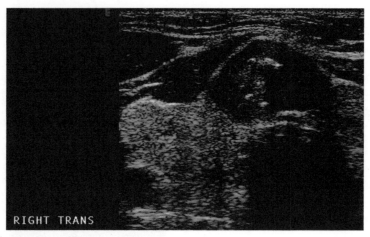

Fig. 7. Microcalcifications in a PTC.

nodules, and found that the sensitivity and specificity of this technique for thyroid cancer diagnosis ranges from 82% to 100% and 81% to 97%, respectively.[31,36,37] Accuracy in one study was approximately 80%.[31] The technique seems to be limited in lesions with coarse calcifications, a significant cystic component, and in differentiating follicular lesions.[31,37] Although the use of this technique remains controversial, lacks standardized measurements for widespread use, and has yet to be prospectively validated, it seems to hold promise in differentiating benign from malignant lesions and may help guide surveillance and selection of nodules for FNA.

ULTRASOUND CHARACTERISTICS OF MALIGNANT LESIONS

Most thyroid nodules are benign, with approximately 10% of nodules representing malignancy.[38] Risk factors for cancer include female gender, advanced age, exposure to ionizing radiation, and a family history of thyroid cancer. Most thyroid cancers are of follicular cell origin, including papillary, follicular, and Hürthle cell carcinoma, collectively called well-differentiated thyroid cancer. Other malignancies such as MTC, anaplastic carcinoma, lymphoma, and metastatic disease are less common.

As mentioned earlier, ultrasound characteristics of thyroid nodules do not offer sufficient specificity to diagnose malignancy. Regardless, ultrasound represents an invaluable tool in identifying thyroid lesions and aids in determining which lesions should undergo further evaluation through biopsy or other investigations. The next sections discuss specific ultrasound characteristics of thyroid malignancies.

PAPILLARY CARCINOMA

PTC is the most common thyroid malignancy and represents 70% to 80% of all thyroid cancers. Female/male ratio is 2:1 and the peak age at diagnosis is 20 to 30 years. Multifocal lesions and regional nodal metastases are common, whereas distant metastases to bone or lung are less common. Local invasion of the larynx, trachea, esophagus, spine, or soft tissues of the neck is seen in only the most aggressive forms of PTC. Prognosis is excellent, with a cure rate up to 90%. Poorer prognosis is associated with large size, advanced patient age, nodal involvement, extrathyroidal spread, male gender, and vascular invasion. Rarely, PTC may degenerate into anaplastic carcinoma.

Ultrasound features typical of PTC include a solid, hypoechoic lesion with microcalcifications (**Fig. 10** and Video 3: PTC in the left thyroid lobe (transverse view). To view video please go to

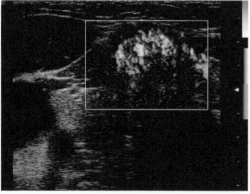

Fig. 8. Increased central blood flow in a papillary carcinoma.

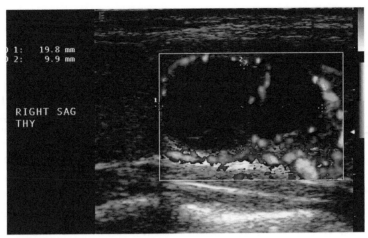

Fig. 9. Follicular adenoma with peripheral blood flow.

www.ultrasound.theclinics.com). Cystic compo-nents may be present within a solid lesion (**Fig. 11**), and although an incomplete halo may be seen, ill-defined margins are more common. Doppler examination may also reveal disorganized hypervascularity. Of these features, microcalcifica-tions may be the most specific for PTC because psammoma bodies are a histopathologic feature considered pathognomonic for PTC; they are composed of tiny laminated, spherical collections of calcium that reflect sound waves and appear as tiny bright foci.

FOLLICULAR CARCINOMA

Follicular carcinoma accounts for approximately 10% of thyroid malignancies. It is more common in older women, has a female/male ratio of 3:1, and has a mean age at diagnosis of 50 years.[39] Unlike PTC, follicular carcinoma is more likely to spread via hematogenous routes, accounting for a higher incidence of distant metastases and poorer prognosis.

Follicular neoplasms, both benign and malig-nant, typically appear as solid, hypoechoic, and homogenous lesions (**Fig. 12**). Cystic components and calcifications are rare and a halo is often seen. Hypervascularity is common and FNA samples are often bloody. The most important prognostic features are whether vascular, extracapsular, and/or local invasion is present. Because follicular adenoma cannot be distinguished cytologically from follicular carcinoma on FNA, the predomi-nance of follicular cells on FNA, especially in sheets or microfollicles, often necessitates an excisional biopsy of the affected lobe.

HÜRTHLE CELL CARCINOMA

The World Health Organization classification of thyroid lesions considers Hürthle cell tumors to

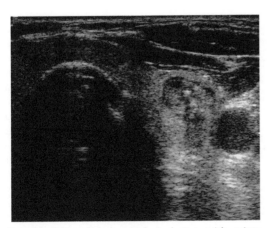

Fig. 10. PTC: solid, hypoechoic lesion with micro-calcifications.

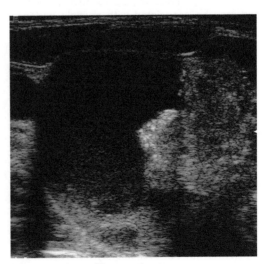

Fig. 11. Cystic papillary carcinoma.

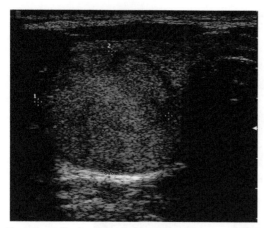

Fig. 12. Follicular neoplasm, appearing as a solid, hypoechoic, and homogenous lesion. This nodule proved to be a follicular adenoma.

be a subtype of follicular cell neoplasm. Approximately 20% of Hürthle cell lesions are malignant and they account for only 3% of thyroid cancers. These tumors behave more aggressively than either PTC or follicular carcinoma, and often present with bilateral and multifocal lesions, with a higher risk of regional lymph node and distant metastasis.

On ultrasound, Hürthle cell tumors are solid, with both hypoechoic and hyperechoic components with an irregular border (**Fig. 13**). Most do not have calcifications or a halo.

MEDULLARY CARCINOMA

MTCs account for 5% of thyroid cancers. They arise from parafollicular C cells, which are primarily concentrated in the superior poles.[39] Women and men are affected equally, and although most cases are spontaneous, up to 30% are familial and may be associated with multiple endocrine

neoplasia (MEN) syndromes type 2A and 2B. MTC occurring in the setting of an MEN syndrome is usually multifocal and bilateral. Spread to regional lymph nodes in the neck and/or mediastinum and hematogenous spread are common.

MTC appears solid and hypoechoic on ultrasound yet frequently has hyperechoic foci, representing both amyloid deposition and calcification (**Fig. 14**). These foci may also appear within affected lymph nodes. As with papillary carcinoma, Doppler examination may reveal disorganized hypervascularity.[40]

ANAPLASTIC CARCINOMA

Anaplastic carcinoma is the most aggressive type of thyroid cancer. Although it accounts for less than 2% of all thyroid cancers, it comprises up to 40% of deaths from thyroid cancer.[41] It is a disease of elderly people, with few cases occurring in patients younger than 50 years. Most anaplastic carcinomas develop in the setting of a preexisting or coexisting thyroid cancer or goiter and may represent malignant transformation of a previously well-differentiated carcinoma. Patients typically present with a rapidly enlarging neck mass associated with pain, voice changes, dysphagia, or dyspnea. Most patients have lymph node involvement at the time of diagnosis.

Ultrasound shows a diffusely hypoechoic lesion, often infiltrating the entire thyroid lobe, with areas of necrosis or ill-defined calcifications (**Fig. 15**). Involved lymph nodes may also have necrotic changes. Invasion into surrounding vessels or soft tissue is often seen.

LYMPHOMA

Lymphoma involving the thyroid gland is rare, accounting for less than 5% of thyroid malignancies.[41] It may be primary or arise as part of

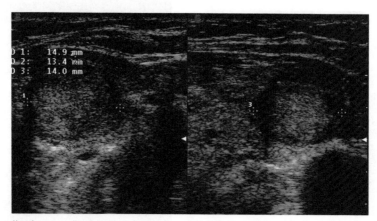

Fig. 13. Hürthle cell adenoma (by histology) that is solid with both hypoechoic and hyperechoic components (*transverse and sagittal views*).

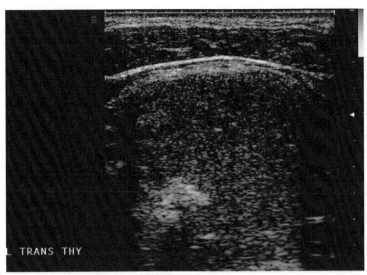

Fig. 14. MTC that appears solid and hypoechoic, yet has hyperechoic foci, representing both amyloid deposition and calcification.

a systemic lymphoma. Women are more often affected and age at diagnosis is usually greater than 50 years. Non-Hodgkin lymphoma is the most common type and is usually associated with a history of Hashimoto thyroiditis. The cytologic diagnosis can be easily mistaken for chronic lymphocytic thyroiditis. The clinical course of thyroid lymphoma may resemble anaplastic carcinoma, with a rapidly enlarging neck mass, regional lymph node enlargement, and symptoms related to compression of the recurrent laryngeal nerve or trachea. However, lymphoma is usually not associated with pain. Local soft-tissue and vascular invasion are both common.

Lymphoma may appear as a focal lesion within a lobe or as a diffuse abnormality involving the entire gland (**Fig. 16**). The involved tissue is usually heterogeneous and hypoechoic and may be mistaken for anaplastic carcinoma. Pseudocysts with posterior enhancement are sometimes seen.

THYROID AS A SITE OF CANCER METASTASES

Metastases to the thyroid gland are uncommon and usually arise from a primary melanoma, breast, lung, or renal cell carcinoma.[39,40] Thyroid metastases usually involve the inferior poles and are homogenous, hypoechoic, and noncalcified.

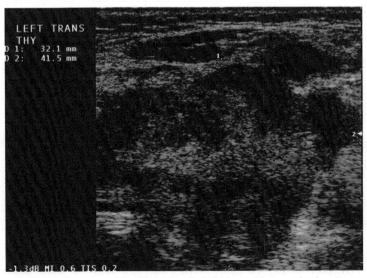

Fig. 15. Anaplastic carcinoma, seen as a diffusely hypoechoic lesion with irregular borders.

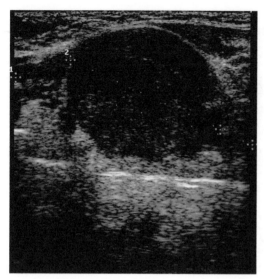

Fig. 16. Lymphoma may appear as a focal heterogeneous and hypoechoic lesion within a background of chronic lymphocytic thyroiditis.

LYMPH NODES

The cervical nodal beds should be evaluated for the presence of abnormally enlarged or otherwise abnormal lymph nodes. Prelaryngeal, pretracheal, and paratracheal (level VI) lymph nodes are a common site of thyroid carcinoma metastasis (Video 4: Left level 6 lymph node metastases from papillary thyroid carcinoma, sometimes visible even in the presence of the thyroid gland - transverse view sweeping inferior to the left thyroid lobe. To view video please go to www.ultrasound. theclinics.com); however, these nodes are often not amenable to adequate ultrasound evaluation because of thyroid gland obstruction. In contrast, ultrasound is useful and sensitive in the pretreatment evaluation of lateral cervical lymph nodes,

and of the central (level VI) compartment after thyroidectomy. Ultrasound is also invaluable in the surveillance for recurrent thyroid cancer. The same ultrasound characteristics that are suggestive of malignancy within a thyroid nodule may be found in cervical lymph node metastases. Several features, including cystic appearance, hyperechoic punctuations, loss of hilum, and peripheral vascularization have been associated with malignancy.[42,43] Enlargement, rounded shape, and irregular or indistinct margins can also be seen (**Fig. 17**).[44]

ULTRASOUND SURVEILLANCE OF BENIGN NODULES

Thyroid nodules that appear benign on both cytology and ultrasound should be clinically followed over time. Although malignant transformation of benign thyroid nodules is believed to be rare, there is a 3% to 5% false-negative rate of FNA. Both the ATA and AACE/AME recommend that cytologically benign thyroid nodules be followed every 6 to 18 months with palpation if easily palpable or with ultrasound if not easily palpable.[1,2] The nodules should undergo repeat FNA if there is evidence for nodule growth, defined as a 20% increase in nodule diameter with a minimum increase in 2 or more dimensions of at least 2 mm.[1]

ROLE OF ULTRASOUND IN THYROID GLAND DISEASES
Graves Disease

Palpable thyroid nodules are found 3 times as frequently in patients with Graves disease compared with the general population, and approximately 17% of these nodules harbor malignancy.[45] A prospective study evaluated patients

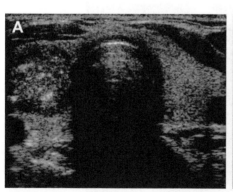
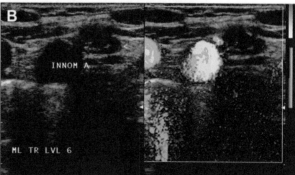

Fig. 17. Similar ultrasound features, including hypoechoic and/or cystic appearance, microcalcifications, and peripheral vascularization can be seen in this primary PTC in the right thyroid lobe (*A*) and within an adjacent low midline level VI lymph node (*B*). The figure shows a scan in a transverse plane, descending through the thyroid and to the suprasternal level VI, where the metastatic node abuts the innominate artery.

with Graves disease with physical examination, ultrasound, and scintigraphy; thyroid nodules were identified in 47%, 16%, and 2% of patients, respectively, and 54% of the nodules identified with ultrasound harbored malignancy.[46] The investigators advocate ultrasound examination of all patients with Graves disease.

Ultrasound features of thyroid glands in patients with Graves disease include heterogeneous tissue with diffuse hypoechogenicity and hypervascularity (**Fig. 18**). The velocity of flow in the inferior thyroid artery is typically increased. Color flow mapping may be useful in selecting the optimal dose of antithyroid medication to achieve a euthyroid state,[47] and may also be predictive of the likelihood of relapse after the withdrawal of antithyroid medications.[48,49]

Multinodular Goiter

The risk of malignancy is similar in patients with multiple nodules compared with those with single nodules.[8] The number of nodules present has not been shown to correlate with risk of malignancy.[33] Each nodule should be evaluated independently. In patients with more then one nodule greater than 1 cm, FNA should be guided by ultrasound characteristics suspicious for malignancy rather than size.[1,2] If multiple enlarged nodules are present and none displays suspicious findings on ultrasound, the largest or most solid and hypoechoic nodules should be considered for sampling and smaller nodules followed with serial ultrasound examinations (Video 5: Transverse sweep through the right lobe of a multinodular goiter. To

view video please go to www.ultrasound.the clinics.com).[1]

Thyroiditis

The rate of malignancy in nodules in patients with Hashimoto thyroiditis is equal to or greater than those in normal thyroid glands.[50,51] The ATA recommends that all patients with an increased level of thyroid-stimulating hormone undergo diagnostic ultrasound.[1] Ultrasound findings include ill-defined hypoechoic areas separated by echogenic septa, with increased or decreased vascularity (**Fig. 19**). Intrathyroid lymphoid tissue accumulates as a result of the autoimmune process in association with thyroid peroxidase antibodies,[52] and patients with Hashimoto thyroiditis have up to a 60-fold increase in the risk of developing lymphoma.[53,54] Chronic lymphocytic thyroiditis is also often associated with central compartment inflammatory lymphadenopathy, which can be difficult to distinguish from small malignant lymphadenopathy.

Thyroid Cysts

Cystic nodules represent approximately 20% of all thyroid nodules.[16] Purely cystic lesions are nearly uniformly benign; however, these comprise only 2% of all cystic lesions.[26] Approximately 15% of cystic nodules represent necrotic papillary cancers and 30% represent hemorrhagic adenomas.[9] Most decrease in size over time or completely disappear.[55] Rates of nondiagnostic FNA are high with cystic lesions, and therefore ultrasound-guided

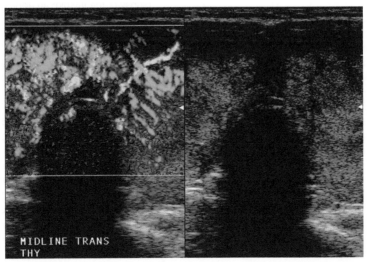

Fig. 18. Thyroid ultrasonography in Graves disease shows thickened heterogeneous parenchyma with diffuse hypoechogenicity and hypervascularity.

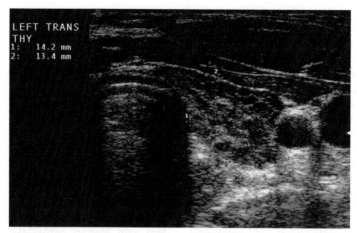

Fig. 19. In late-stage Hashimoto thyroiditis, the thyroid is diffusely heterogeneous and atrophic.

FNA is recommended to ensure sampling of the solid component.[1]

SUMMARY: ULTRASOUND AS A TOOL FOR OTOLARYNGOLOGISTS

Thyroid ultrasonography has proved to be an invaluable, first-line tool in the evaluation, management, and treatment of a variety of thyroid disorders. Its indications and uses span both benign and malignant diseases, and continue to expand with improvements in technology. A variety of physicians find benefit by incorporating thyroid ultrasonography into their clinical and operative practice.

REFERENCES

1. Cooper DS, Doherty GM, Haugen BR, et al. Revised American Thyroid Association management guidelines for patients with thyroid nodules and differentiated thyroid cancer. Thyroid 2009;19:1167–214.
2. Gharib H, Papini E, Valcavi R, et al. American Association of Clinical Endocrinologists and Associazione Medici Endocrinologi medical guidelines for clinical practice for the diagnosis and management of thyroid nodules. Endocr Pract 2006;12:63–102.
3. Thijs LG. Diagnostic ultrasound in clinical thyroid investigation. J Clin Endocrinol Metab 1971;32:709–16.
4. Rosen IB, Walfish PG, Miskin M. The application of ultrasound to the study of thyroid enlargement: management of 450 cases. Arch Surg 1975;110:940–4.
5. Spencer R, Brown MC, Annis D. Ultrasonic scanning of the thyroid gland as a guide to the treatment of the clinically solitary nodule. Br J Surg 1977;64:841–6.
6. Lees WR, Vahl SP, Watson LR, et al. The role of ultrasound scanning in the diagnosis of thyroid swellings. Br J Surg 1978;65:681–4.
7. Mortensen JD, Woolner LB, Bennett WA. Gross and microscopic findings in clinically normal thyroid glands. J Clin Endocrinol Metab 1955;15:1270–80.
8. Marqusee E, Benson CB, Frates MC, et al. Usefulness of ultrasonography in the management of nodular thyroid disease. Ann Intern Med 2000;133:696–700.
9. Mazzaferri EL. Management of a solitary thyroid nodule. N Engl J Med 1993;328:553–9.
10. Tunbridge WM, Evered DC, Hall R, et al. The spectrum of thyroid disease in a community: the Whickham survey. Clin Endocrinol (Oxf) 1977;7:481–93.
11. Gharib H, Goellner JR. Fine-needle aspiration biopsy of the thyroid: an appraisal. Ann Intern Med 1993;118:282–9.
12. Cesur M, Corapcioglu D, Bulut S, et al. Comparison of palpation-guided fine-needle aspiration biopsy to ultrasound-guided fine-needle aspiration biopsy in the evaluation of thyroid nodules. Thyroid 2006;16:555–61.
13. Koike E, Yamashita H, Noguchi S, et al. Effect of combining ultrasonography and ultrasound-guided fine-needle aspiration biopsy findings for the diagnosis of thyroid nodules. Eur J Surg 2001;167:656–61.
14. Hatada T, Okada K, Ishii H, et al. Evaluation of ultrasound-guided fine-needle aspiration biopsy for thyroid nodules. Am J Surg 1998;175:133–6.
15. Takashima S, Fukuda H, Kobayashi T. Thyroid nodules: clinical effect of ultrasound-guided fine-needle aspiration biopsy. J Clin Ultrasound 1994;22:535–42.
16. Morris LF, Ragavendra N, Yeh MW. Evidence-based assessment of the role of ultrasonography in the

management of benign thyroid nodules. World J Surg 2008;32:1253–63.

17. Cappelli C, Castellano M, Pirola I, et al. The predictive value of ultrasound findings in the management of thyroid nodules. QJM 2007;100:29–35.

18. Kim EK, Park CS, Chung WY, et al. New sonographic criteria for recommending fine-needle aspiration biopsy of nonpalpable solid nodules of the thyroid. AJR Am J Roentgenol 2002;178:687–91.

19. Hagag P, Strauss S, Weiss M. Role of ultrasound-guided fine-needle aspiration biopsy in evaluation of nonpalpable thyroid nodules. Thyroid 1998;8:989–95.

20. Nam-Goong IS, Kim HY, Gong G, et al. Ultrasonography-guided fine-needle aspiration of thyroid incidentaloma: correlation with pathological findings. Clin Endocrinol (Oxf) 2004;60:21–8.

21. Papini E, Guglielmi R, Bianchini A, et al. Risk of malignancy in nonpalpable thyroid nodules: predictive value of ultrasound and color-Doppler features. J Clin Endocrinol Metab 2002;87:1941–6.

22. Ultrasonography of the Thyroid. Thyroid disease manager. Chapter 6C. Available at: http://www.thyroidmanager.org. Accessed November 20, 2009.

23. Baskin HJ. Thyroid ultrasound and ultrasound-guided FNA biopsy. Norwell (MA): Kluwer Academic Publishers; 2000.

24. Koike E, Noguchi S, Yamashita H, et al. Ultrasonographic characteristics of thyroid nodules: prediction of malignancy. Arch Surg 2001;136:334–7.

25. Leenhardt L, Menegaux F, Franc B, et al. Selection of patients with solitary thyroid nodules for operation. Eur J Surg 2002;168:236–41.

26. Frates MC, Benson CB, Doubilet PM, et al. Prevalence and distribution of carcinoma in patients with solitary and multiple thyroid nodules on sonography. J Clin Endocrinol Metab 2006;91:3411–7.

27. Moon WJ, Jung SL, Lee JH, et al. Benign and malignant thyroid nodules: US differentiation–multicenter retrospective study. Radiology 2008;247:762–70.

28. Bonavita JA, Mayo J, Babb J, et al. Pattern recognition of benign nodules at ultrasound of the thyroid: which nodules can be left alone? AJR Am J Roentgenol 2009;193:207–13.

29. Kang HW, No JH, Chung JH, et al. Prevalence, clinical and ultrasonographic characteristics of thyroid incidentalomas. Thyroid 2004;14:29–33.

30. Seiberling KA, Dutra JC, Grant T, et al. Role of intrathyroidal calcifications detected on ultrasound as a marker of malignancy. Laryngoscope 2004;114:1753–7.

31. Asteria C, Giovanardi A, Pizzocaro A, et al. US-elastography in the differential diagnosis of benign and malignant thyroid nodules. Thyroid 2008;18:523–31.

32. Iannuccilli JD, Cronan JJ, Monchik JM. Risk for malignancy of thyroid nodules as assessed by sonographic criteria: the need for biopsy. J Ultrasound Med 2004;23:1455–64.

33. Chammas MC, Gerhard R, de Oliveira IR, et al. Thyroid nodules: evaluation with power Doppler and duplex Doppler ultrasound. Otolaryngol Head Neck Surg 2005;132:874–82.

34. Miyakawa M, Onoda N, Etoh M, et al. Diagnosis of thyroid follicular carcinoma by the vascular pattern and velocimetric parameters using high resolution pulsed and power Doppler ultrasonography. Endocr J 2005;52:207–12.

35. Chaturvedi P, Insana MF, Hall TJ. Ultrasonic and elasticity imaging to model disease-induced changes in soft-tissue structure. Med Image Anal 1998;2:325–38.

36. Rago T, Santini F, Scutari M, et al. Elastography: new developments in ultrasound for predicting malignancy in thyroid nodules. J Clin Endocrinol Metab 2007;92:2917–22.

37. Lyshchik A, Higashi T, Asato R, et al. Thyroid gland tumor diagnosis at US elastography. Radiology 2005;237:202–11.

38. Mandel SJ. A 64-year-old woman with a thyroid nodule. JAMA 2004;292:2632–42.

39. Cummings CW, Haughey B, Thomas JR, et al. Cummings otolaryngology – head and neck surgery. 4th edition. St Louis (MO): Mosby; 2005.

40. Ahuja A. Practical head and neck ultrasound. London: Greenwich Medical Media; 2000.

41. Green LD, Mack L, Pasieka JL. Anaplastic thyroid cancer and primary thyroid lymphoma: a review of these rare thyroid malignancies. J Surg Oncol 2006;94:725–36.

42. Leboulleux S, Girard E, Rose M, et al. Ultrasound criteria of malignancy for cervical lymph nodes in patients followed up for differentiated thyroid cancer. J Clin Endocrinol Metab 2007;92:3590–4.

43. Rosario PW, de Faria S, Bicalho L, et al. Ultrasonographic differentiation between metastatic and benign lymph nodes in patients with papillary thyroid carcinoma. J Ultrasound Med 2005;24:1385–9.

44. Orloff LA. Head and neck ultrasonography. San Diego (CA): Plural Publishing; 2008.

45. Belfiore A, Russo D, Vigneri R, et al. Graves' disease, thyroid nodules and thyroid cancer. Clin Endocrinol (Oxf) 2001;55:711–8.

46. Cappelli C, Pirola I, De Martino E, et al. The role of imaging in Graves' disease: a cost-effectiveness analysis. Eur J Radiol 2008;65:99–103.

47. Saleh A, Furst G, Feldkamp J, et al. Estimation of antithyroid drug dose in Graves' disease: value of quantification of thyroid blood flow with color duplex sonography. Ultrasound Med Biol 2001;27:1137–41.

48. Saleh A, Cohnen M, Furst G, et al. Prediction of relapse after antithyroid drug therapy of Graves' disease: value of color Doppler sonography. Exp Clin Endocrinol Diabetes 2004;112:510–3.

49. Varsamidis K, Varsamidou E, Mavropoulos G. Doppler ultrasonography in predicting relapse of hyperthyroidism in Graves' disease. Acta Radiol 2000;41:45–8.

50. Singh B, Shaha AR, Trivedi H, et al. Coexistent Hashimoto's thyroiditis with papillary thyroid carcinoma: impact on presentation, management, and outcome. Surgery 1999;126:1070–6 [discussion: 1076–7].

51. Repplinger D, Bargren A, Zhang YW, et al. Is Hashimoto's thyroiditis a risk factor for papillary thyroid cancer? J Surg Res 2008;150:49–52.

52. Thieblemont C, Mayer A, Dumontet C, et al. Primary thyroid lymphoma is a heterogeneous disease. J Clin Endocrinol Metab 2002;87:105–11.

53. Kato I, Tajima K, Suchi T, et al. Chronic thyroiditis as a risk factor of B-cell lymphoma in the thyroid gland. Jpn J Cancer Res 1985;76:1085–90.

54. Holm LE, Blomgren H, Lowhagen T. Cancer risks in patients with chronic lymphocytic thyroiditis. N Engl J Med 1985;312:601–4.

55. Kuma K, Matsuzuka F, Yokozawa T, et al. Fate of untreated benign thyroid nodules: results of long-term follow-up. World J Surg 1994;18:495–8 [discussion: 499].

Techniques for Parathyroid Localization with Ultrasound

Lisa Lee, MD, David L. Steward, MD*

KEYWORDS

- Parathyroid adenoma • Parathyroid localization
- Ultrasonography

PARATHYROID WORKUP

Four-gland parathyroid exploration has been the gold standard for parathyroid surgery until recently. Emphasis is now placed on minimally invasive and focused parathyroidectomy. Given this objective, there is a need for sensitive and accurate localization of parathyroid pathology. Effective imaging techniques are instrumental in achieving these ends, particularly in the midst of heightened awareness of cost containment.

A thorough medical workup identifies the cause underlying hypercalcemia in the vast majority of patients. Hyperparathyroidism accounts for most cases of hypercalcemia and is categorized as primary, secondary, or tertiary. Primary hyperparathyroidism is the most common cause of hypercalcemia, affecting an estimated 0.2% to 0.5% of the US population. There are approximately 100,000 new cases each year.[1] One in 500 women and one in 2000 men usually in their fifties to seventies are affected.[2] Clinical manifestations of hypercalcemia include fatigue, hypertension, bone pain, muscle weakness, renal stones, peptic ulcers, and psychiatric illness.[2,3] Laboratory abnormalities include hypercalcemia, hypophosphatemia, elevated parathyroid hormone levels, and increased urine calcium excretion. Secondary hyperparathyroidism is usually found in patients with renal insufficiency marked by hypocalcemia and hyperphosphatemia or in the setting of vitamin D deficiency. Tertiary hyperparathyroidism occurs with the development of autonomously hyperfunctioning parathyroid glands of secondary hyperparathyroidism with resultant hypercalcemia.[4–7]

Primary hyperparathyroidism may be sporadic or hereditary, with sporadic being much more common. Spontaneous primary hyperparathyroidism is most often due to solitary parathyroid adenomas (85 to 90%), 4-gland hyperplasia (10 to 15%) or multiple adenomas, or asymmetric hyperplasia (2 to 3%) but rarely due to parathyroid carcinoma (<1%).[3,8–10] Hereditary primary hyperparathyroidism may be isolated, associated with jaw tumor syndrome or other endocrine neoplasia. In hereditary primary hyperparathyroidism, multigland disease (multiple endocrine neoplasia 1 or 2a) is the rule rather than the exception.[11]

Identification and localization of parathyroid adenomas is crucial for selective parathyroid surgery. Previously, the predominant localization technique involved sestamibi scanning. Its limitations have prompted investigations for more effective tools, including ultrasound technology. Unlike sestamibi scanning, ultrasonography offers more precise anatomic localization with concomitant facilitation of surgical planning.

This article was previously published in the December 2010 issue of *Otolaryngologic Clinics of North America*.
Department of Otolaryngology-Head and Neck Surgery, University of Cincinnati Medical Center, Medical Sciences Building, Room 6507, 231 Albert Sabin Way, Cincinnati, OH 45267-0582, USA
* Corresponding author.
E-mail address: david.steward@uc.edu

Ultrasound Clin 7 (2012) 211–218
doi:10.1016/j.cult.2011.12.005

ULTRASONOGRAPHY IN THE PARATHYROID WORKUP

In the setting of primary hyperparathyroidism, one study found that ultrasonography had a sensitivity, specificity, and positive predictive value of 60%, 91%, and 92%, respectively, in detecting adenomas.[12] In the authors' experience of surgically proven adenomas, ultrasound sensitivity was 90%, better than sestamibi (70%).[13] Ultrasonography is a much less sensitive tool for identifying hyperplasia.[14] In the setting of secondary hyperparathyroidism, ultrasound had a sensitivity of 60% and accuracy of 64% in localizing enlarged parathyroid glands, missing as many as 30% of patients with multigland disease.[12,15] Furthermore, patients with negative localization by scintigraphy and ultrasound were more likely to have 4-gland hyperplasia.

The accuracy of ultrasonography is also affected by thyroid disease, because its sensitivity dropped from 100% to 84% to 93% and positive predictive value decreased from 100% to 84%.[16–18] Nodular thyroid disease may also contribute to false-positive or negative results. Infrathyroidal lymph nodes associated with thyroiditis may result in a false-positive interpretation as inferior adenomas. Decreased sensitivity is often a consequence of poor echogenic differentiation of parathyroid tissue.

ANATOMY & EMBRYOLOGY

Most individuals have 4 parathyroid glands (80%), 2 superior and 2 inferior. Supernumerary fifth or sixth glands may be found in 13% to 25% of the population, whereas 3% to 5% of the population has fewer than 4 parathyroid glands.[4,19–22] Approximately 1% to 3% of parathyroid glands are ectopic.[19,22]

The superior parathyroid glands arise from the fourth branchial pouch. They descend the neck in an inferoposterior direction to reside posterior to the recurrent laryngeal nerve, a sixth arch derivative. Most superior parathyroid glands are located posterior to the middle or upper portion of the thyroid gland in the vicinity of the cricothyroid junction. Less commonly, they may be located inferior to the midportion of the thyroid lobe (4%) or above the superior pole of the thyroid gland (3%). Occasionally, superior parathyroid glands may migrate toward the tracheoesophageal groove or the posterior mediastinum. Such ectopic adenomas account for less than 3% and may be found in the retropharyngeal, retroesophageal, posterior paratracheal, or intrathyroidal spaces.[19,22–26]

The inferior parathyroid glands arise from the third branchial pouch. They descend the neck in an inferoanterior direction, often in close association with the thymus, and eventually reside anterior to the recurrent laryngeal nerve. Because the inferior parathyroid glands travel a greater distance, there is more variability in their final position. They may be found anywhere from the hyoid bone to the pericardium. More often, they are located inferior or just posterior to the lower pole of the thyroid, near the inferior thyroid artery (45%–60%).[19,22,23,25,26]

Ectopic inferior parathyroid glands may be found in the cervical thymus (26%), anterosuperior mediastinum within the thymus (2%), or inferior to the thymus deep in the mediastinum (0.2%). Alternatively, the inferior parathyroid glands may fail to adequately descend and consequently remain cephalad to the superior glands. Ectopic glands within the carotid sheath may be surrounded by thymic fat. They may also be recognized within the inferior pole of the thyroid gland.[21,27–29]

SONOGRAPHIC APPEARANCE OF THE PARATHYROID GLANDS

Normal parathyroid glands are rarely visualized, because of their small size and insufficient acoustic difference from surrounding tissue. The average size of a normal parathyroid gland is $5 \times 3 \times 1$ mm, with a range of 2 to 12 mm. Each gland usually weighs an average of 40 mg with a range of 10 to 78 mg.[14,22,23,25] In contrast, parathyroid adenomas, hyperplasia, and carcinomas exhibit a relatively hypoechogenic pattern, because of their compact cellularity relative to thyroid tissue.[18] Hyperplastic glands in primary hyperparathyroidism are often 2 to 4 times larger than normal. However, hyperplastic parathyroids are difficult to detect unless they exhibit a significant increase in total gland volume. Microcalcifications may be present in hyperplasia, particularly in patients with secondary hyperparathyroidism.[14] Enlarged parathyroids with indistinct borders suggest a carcinoma.[30–32]

Parathyroid adenomas are usually well-circumscribed ovoid, bilobed, polygonal, triangular, or longitudinal in shape. They tend to be solid and homogenously hypoechoic relative to echogenic thyroid tissue.[9,10,19,20,33] Overall, the ability to detect a parathyroid adenoma is a function of its size. The smaller the adenoma, the more difficult the task of localizing it radiographically. The lower limit of detection was reported to be 4 to 8 mm, with a 90% accurate rate of diagnosis in glands weighing more than 500 mg, although the authors often detect small adenomas down to 100 to 200 mg.[13,34,35] The average mass of parathyroid adenomas is 10 times greater than normal parathyroid glands.[36–38] Rarely, cystic changes or calcifications may be seen in adenomas undergoing complete or partial cystic degeneration.[33,39–42] Seldom encountered, lipoadenomas appear hyperechoic because of increased fat content within the parathyroid adenoma.[43]

SONOGRAPHIC TECHNIQUE

To begin the ultrasonographic examination, the patient is placed in a comfortable, semireclined position facing midline, with the neck mildly extended. Neck extension allows slight elevation of mediastinal structures out of the thoracic inlet and may be exaggerated for mediastinal imaging. In most patients, a high frequency linear transducer may be used (8 to 15 MHz). Examination of larger patients may require a lower frequency to allow adequate sonographic penetration.

The proper frequency setting should allow optimal spatial resolution while also enabling adequate tissue penetration to visualize deep structures, such as the prevertebral musculature. Increasing the far-field or overall gain may also improve detection of deep parathyroid glands by facilitating the sonographic difference between prevertebral musculature and parathyroid tissue.[7,21,44–48]

Ultrasonographic examination ideally follows a routine pathway, focusing on one side of the neck at a time in a slow and deliberate fashion. Initial evaluation involves the central neck compartment, focusing between the carotid arteries laterally and trachea medially. Starting in the transverse plane at the level of the innominate vessels inferiorly, scanning can progress superiorly to the superior pole of the thyroid or hyoid. The transducer is then moved in a lateral to medial direction for longitudinal scanning. Although longitudinal scanning is initially more challenging, it is necessary to corroborate abnormalities detected in the transverse plane and to detect adenomas missed with transverse scanning.

Skin and subcutaneous fat is first encountered by sound waves. Beneath these layers, the strap muscles (sternohyoid, omohyoid, and sternothyroid) centrally and sternocleidomastoid muscle laterally are visualized.

Muscle tissue may be distinguished by its fibrillar hypoechoic appearance compared with the echogenic texture of thyroid tissue. The thyroid gland may be assessed for nodules and microcalcifications among other features.

The esophagus may be found to the left side of the trachea. It has a hypoechoic peripheral muscular layer and an echogenic central mucosa. It may be better identified on dynamic imaging while observing the patient swallow. The prevertebral musculature is seen posterior to the thyroid gland.

Laterally in the neck, the contents of the carotid sheath may be seen adjacent to the thyroid gland. A distinction between the artery and vein can be made based on the compressibility of venous structures and more anterior and lateral position of the internal jugular vein.

The central neck is first evaluated for orthotopic parathyroid glands, with particular attention to the common locations aforementioned. The superior gland is commonly found posterior to the middle third of the thyroid gland and sometimes in the trachea-esophageal groove, (**Fig. 1**) demonstrate

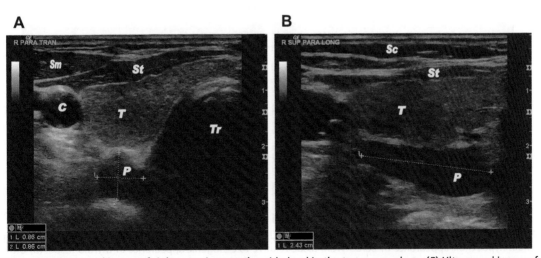

Fig. 1. (*A*) Ultrasound image of right superior parathyroid gland in the transverse plane. (*B*) Ultrasound image of right superior parathyroid gland in the longitudinal plane. C, Carotid artery; P, Parathyroid gland; P, Parathyroid gland; Sm, Sternocleidomastoid muscle; St, Strap muscle; T, Thyroid gland; Tr, Trachea; Sc, Subcutaneous tissue; St, Strap muscle; T, Thyroid gland.

the location of an orthotopic superior parathyroid gland. The inferior gland usually lies near the inferior pole of the thyroid gland, (**Fig. 2**) demonstrate the location of an orthotopic inferior parathyroid gland.

If an adenoma is not identified after scanning the central neck in the transverse and longitudinal planes, then a systematic search for common ectopic locations is conducted. Common ectopic locations for superior parathyroid glands are retroesophageal, deep inferior mediastinum, and, occasionally, posterior intrathyroidal.

Common ectopic locations for inferior parathyroid glands are inferior intrathyroidal, intrathymic, carotid sheath, or anterior mediastinum. Intrathyroidal parathyroid glands may be differentiated from thyroid nodules or thyroid parenchyma by their relatively hypoechoic signal; however, differentiation may require ultrasound-guided fine-needle aspiration (FNA) for cytology, staining, and parathyroid hormone assay of needle-wash contents.

An enlarged gland in the paraesophageal region may pop into view by having patients turn their head away from the side being examined and then swallowing. A hypoechoic mass will be visible along a backdrop of a longitudinally directed muscle. Also, aiming the transducer medially aids in the evaluation of the retrotracheal or paratracheal region; however, retrotracheal ectopic glands may be difficult to detect because of the poor acoustic window caused by the tracheal air column.

A more lateral position of the transducer may decrease the shadow artifact related to the carotid artery and trachea, when examining the central compartment posterior to the carotid artery and trachea.

Tilting the transducer probe is a good adjunct technique to moving the transducer during scanning. To assist in visualization of deeply inferior parathyroid glands, the patient swallows while the ultrasound probe is aimed inferiorly underneath the clavicles. Despite swallowing maneuvers, visualization of mediastinal glands is often difficult because of poor penetration by sound waves.[21,44–47,49,50]

The distinction between superior and inferior parathyroid glands can be occasionally difficult. The key distinguishing feature is based on embryologic origin. Superior parathyroid glands lie in a deeper plane than inferior parathyroid glands. Superior parathyroid glands lie posterior to the plane of the recurrent laryngeal nerve. The posterior surface of the common carotid artery or the inferior thyroid artery may be used as surrogate markers for the recurrent laryngeal nerve. Hence, an adenoma located entirely deep to these landmarks is most likely a superior parathyroid gland, even if located more inferiorly from its usual orthotopic location.

DIFFERENTIATING PARATHYROID GLANDS

Any potential candidate for a parathyroid adenoma must be confirmed in 2 views, in longitudinal and transverse planes, to avoid the pitfalls of false-positive examinations. Normal anatomic structures may be mistaken for parathyroid tissue. Thyroid nodules, enlarged lymph nodes, esophagus, longus

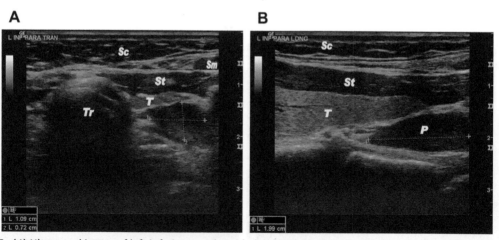

Fig. 2. (*A*) Ultrasound image of left inferior parathyroid gland in the transverse plane. Note the relative homogenous hypoechoic appearance of parathyroid tissue relative to echogenic appearance of thyroid tissue. (*B*) Ultrasound image of left inferior parathyroid gland in the longitudinal plane. Note the elongated, relative homogenous hypoechoic appearance of parathyroid tissue relative to echogenic appearance of thyroid tissue. P, Parathyroid gland; Sc, subcutaneous tissue; Sm, sternocleidomastoid muscle; St, strap muscle; Tr, trachea; T, thyroid gland.

colli, and small vessels may be inadvertently mistaken for parathyroid lesions.[51]

Thyroid gland abnormalities may obscure adequate visualization of parathyroid pathology. The sensitivity of high-frequency ultrasound decreases in patients with thyroid nodules compared with patients without thyroid pathology, reducing from 85% to 100% sensitivity to 47% to 84%.[12,17,52,53] In the setting of multinodular goiter, parathyroid adenomas may be overlooked because of poor sonographic penetration, dispersion of the sound waves, or difficulty distinguishing the parathyroid capsule because of the goitrous contour. Alternatively, thyroid nodules may be mistaken for parathyroid adenomas, particularly if they are located posteriorly on the thyroid capsule, (Fig. 3) demonstrates a thyroid nodule which may be mistaken for a parathyroid gland.[54,55] Swallowing maneuvers sometimes help differentiate extrathyroidal adenomas from the thyroid gland.

Lymph nodes may be mistaken for adenomas because of their size, location, and appearance, especially in the setting of thyroiditis. Distinguishing between lymph node and parathyroid gland may be more difficult in an older patient, because parathyroid glands tend to accumulate more fat and hence take on a more echogenic appearance.

Prevertebral muscles, veins, or esophagus may be mistaken for adenomas if scanned only in a transverse fashion.[9,56] On transverse view, the esophagus may be mistaken for a posterior parathyroid on the left side. However, a longitudinal view would show its tubular appearance. Peristalsis may also be demonstrated on longitudinal view. The longus colli muscle can be more definitively identified on longitudinal scanning.

In addition to transverse and longitudinal gray-scale sonographic views, graded compression and color Doppler features may be occasionally useful supplementary tools. Graded compression of superficial tissue, such as subcutaneous fat and neck musculature, helps image patients with thick necks. It also may discern small adenomas (<1 cm) from surrounding tissue, particularly in the tracheoesophageal groove or along the longus colli.[44] Color Doppler provides information that aids in differentiating parathyroid glands from lymph nodes and thyroid nodules.[27,57] Its use was found to improve sensitivity of parathyroid adenoma detection from 73% to 83%.[46] Color Doppler ultrasound may help identify adenomas by determining the presence of an asymmetric, arclike peripheral hypervascularity.[10,18,45–47,49] In contrast, lymph nodes have a distinct hyperechogenic fatty hilum with a central hilar branching vascular flow pattern. This represents a key distinction, because parathyroid adenomas have a feeding artery with a polar insertion on the long axis.[18,45–47,58]

ULTRASONOGRAPHY SHORTCOMINGS

Ultrasonography as a diagnostic tool is highly dependent on operator skill and patient factors. It also requires a high degree of familiarity with cervical anatomy and knowledge of relative echogenicity of various tissues. Successful ultrasonography requires familiarity with the ultrasound machine, including the use of varying frequencies, gain manipulation, graded compression, and color Doppler. In experienced hands, 70% to 90% of enlarged parathyroid glands can be located.[2,13,56,59] Patient body mass index and neck thickness affect penetration of sound waves.[35] Concomitant thyroid disease makes evaluation of parathyroids more challenging. Limited sound-wave resolution leads to inability to reliably detect small parathyroid glands and to mistake lymph nodes for parathyroid glands.

ULTRASOUND APPLIED TO PARATHYROID PATHOLOGY

Ultrasonography provides cost-effective, convenient, and accurate localization of enlarged parathyroid glands in the vast majority of patients with hyperparathyroidism in conjunction with functional sestamibi scanning. Unlike sestamibi scanning, computed tomography, or other imaging technologies, ultrasonography provides dynamic imaging in the hands of the surgeon who has intimate knowledge of cervical anatomy. The knowledge of exact gland location allows the surgeon to focus tissue

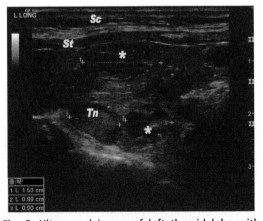

Fig. 3. Ultrasound image of left thyroid lobe with multiple thyroid nodules in the longitudinal plane. The posterior Tn resembles a parathyroid gland. Note the heterogenous appearance of thyroid nodules (*). Sc, subcutaneous tissue; St, strap muscle; Tn, thyroid nodule; *, thyroid nodule.

exploration and consequently decrease chances of injury to significant structures. Particularly with the advent of intraoperative parathyroid hormone levels, focused minimally invasive parathyroidectomy leads to decreased operative time and reduced morbidity as compared with traditional 4-gland exploration.[56,60,61] Novel applications of parathyroid ultrasonography have also evolved to include ultrasound-guided FNA of suspected intrathyroidal parathyroid glands.[16,39,54,62] Also, percutaneous ethanol ablation of hyperplastic parathyroid glands has been applied to chronic dialysis patients.[63] Ultrasound technology applied to parathyroid pathology facilitates directed surgical therapy and minimally invasive applications and consequently holds great promise as a tool that enables cost-effective and advanced patient care.

REFERENCES

1. Zanocco K, Angelos P, Sturgeon C. Cost-effectiveness analysis of parathyroidectomy for asymptomatic primary hyperparathyroidism. Surgery 2006; 140(6):874–81.
2. Uden P, Chan A, Duy QY, et al. Primary hyperparathyroidism in younger and older patients: symptoms and outcome of surgery. World J Surg 1992;16: 791–7.
3. Ruda JM, Hollenbeak CS, Stack BC Jr. A systematic review of the diagnosis and treatment of primary hyperparathyroidism from 1995 to 2003. Otolaryngol Head Neck Surg 2005;132:359–72.
4. Kaplan EL, Yashiro T, Gslti G. Primary hyperparathyroidism in the 1990's. Ann Surg 1992;215:300–17.
5. Pham TH, Sterioff S, Mullan BP, et al. Sensitivity and utility of parathyroid scintigraphy in patients with primary versus secondary and tertiary hyperparathyroidism. World J Surg 2006;30(3):327–32.
6. Ahmad R, Hammond JM. Primary, secondary, and tertiary hyperparathyroidism. Otolaryngol Clin North Am 2004;37(4):701–13.
7. Kamaya A, Quon A, Jeffrey RB. Sonography of the abnormal parathyroid gland. Ultrasound Q 2006; 22(4):253–62.
8. Kebebew E. Predictors of single-gland vs multigland parathyroid disease in primary hyperparathyroidism: a simple and accurate scoring model. Arch Surg 2006;141(8):777–82.
9. Hopkins CR, Reading CC. Thyroid and parathyroid imaging. Semin Ultrasound CT MR 1995;16(4): 279–95.
10. Solbiati L, Osti V, Cova L, et al. Ultrasound of thyroid, parathyroid glands and neck lymph nodes. Eur Radiol 2001;11(12):2411–24.
11. Muhr C, Ljunghall S, Akerstrom G, et al. Screening for multiple endocrine neoplasia syndrome (type 1) in patients with primary hyperparathyroidism. Clin Endocrinol 1984;20:153–62.
12. Sukan A, Reyhan M, Aydin M, et al. Preoperative evaluation of hyperparathyroidism: the role of dual-phase parathyroid scintigraphy and ultrasound imaging. Ann Nucl Med 2008;22(2):123–31.
13. Steward DL, Danielson GP, Afman CE, et al. Parathyroid adenoma localization: surgeon-performed ultrasound versus sestamibi. Laryngoscope 2006; 116(8):1380–4.
14. Mollerup CL, Bollerslev J, Blichert-Toft M. Primary hyperparathyroidism: incidence and clinical and biochemical characteristics—a demographic study. Eur J Surg 1994;160:485–9.
15. Bhansali A, Masoodi SR, Bhadada S, et al. Ultrasonography in detection of single and multiple abnormal parathyroid glands in primary hyperparathyroidism: comparison with radionuclide scintigraphy and surgery. Clin Endocrinol (Oxf) 2006;65(3):340–5.
16. Erbil Y, Salmaslioğlu A, Kabul E, et al. Use of preoperative parathyroid fine-needle aspiration and parathormone assay in the primary hyperparathyroidism with concomitant thyroid nodules. Am J Surg 2007; 193(6):665–71.
17. Erbil Y, Barbaros U, Yanik BT, et al. Impact of gland morphology and concomitant thyroid nodules on preoperative localization of parathyroid adenomas. Laryngoscope 2006;116(4):580–5.
18. Gilat H, Cohen M, Feinmesser R, et al. Minimally invasive procedure for resection of a parathyroid adenoma: the role of preoperative high-resolution ultrasonography. J Clin Ultrasound 2005;33(6):283–7.
19. Wang CA. The anatomic basis of parathyroid surgery. Ann Surg 1976;183:271–5.
20. Reading CC, Charboneau JW, James EM, et al. High-resolution parathyroid sonography. AJR Am J Roentgenol 1982;139:539.
21. Gooding GA. Sonography of the thyroid and parathyroid. Radiol Clin North Am 1993;31:967.
22. Akerstrom G, Malmaeus J, Bergstrom R. Surgical anatomy of human parathyroid glands. Surgery 1984;95:14.
23. Mansberger AR, Wei JP. Surgical embryology and anatomy of the thyroid and parathyroid glands. Surg Clin North Am 1993;73:727.
24. Weller GLJ. Development of the thyroid, parathyroid and thymus glands in man. Contrib Embryol 1933; 24:93.
25. Grimelius L, Bondeson L. Histopathological diagnosis of parathyroid diseases. Pathol Res Pract 1995;191:353–65.
26. Kang YS, Rosen K, Clark OH, et al. Localization of abnormal parathyroid glands of the mediastinum with MR imaging. Radiology 1993;189(1):137–41.
27. Thompson NW, Eckhauser FE, Harness JK. The anatomy of primary hyperparathyroidism. Surgery 1982;92:814.

28. Edis AJ, Purnell DC, van Heerden JA. The unde-scended "parathymus". An occasional cause of failed neck exploration for hyperparathyroidism. Ann Surg 1979;190:64.

29. Edis AJ. Surgical anatomy and technique of neck exploration for primary hyperparathyroidism. Surg Clin North Am 1977;57:495.

30. Edmonson GR, Charboneau JW, James EM, et al. Parathyroid carcinoma: high-frequency sonographic features. Radiology 1986;161:65–7.

31. Smith JF, Coombs RRH. Histological diagnosis of carcinoma of the parathyroid gland. J Clin Pathol 1984;37:1370–8.

32. Kinoshita Y, Fukase M, Uchihashi M, et al. Signifi-cance of preoperative use of ultrasonography in parathyroid neoplasms: comparison of sonographic textures with histologic findings. J Clin Ultrasound 1985;13(7):457–60.

33. Randel SB, Gooding GA, Clark OH, et al. Parathyroid variants: US evaluation. Radiology 1987;165(1):191–4.

34. Kawata R, Kotetsu L, Takamaki A, et al. Ultrasonog-raphy for preoperative localization of enlarged para-thyroid glands in secondary hyperparathyroidism. Auris Nasus Larynx 2009;36(4):461–5.

35. Berber E, Parikh RT, Ballem N, et al. Factors contrib-uting to negative parathyroid localization: an anal-ysis of 1000 patients. Surgery 2008;144(1):74–9.

36. Soon PS, Delbridge LW, Sywak MS, et al. Surgeon performed ultrasound facilitates minimally invasive parathyroidectomy by the focused lateral mini-incision approach. World J Surg 2008;32:766–71.

37. Yao K, Singer FR, Roth SI, et al. Weight of normal para-thyroid glands in patients with parathyroid adenomas. J Clin Endocrinol Metab 2004;89:3208–13.

38. Tresoldi S, Pompili G, Maiolino R, et al. Primary hyperparathyroidism: can ultrasonography be the only preoperative diagnostic procedure? Radiol Med 2009;114:1159–72.

39. Silverman JF, Yhazanie PG, Norris HT, et al. Parathy-roid hormone (PTH) assay of parathyroid cysts examined by fine-needle aspiration biopsy. Am J Clin Pathol 1986;86:776–80.

40. Graif M, Itzchak Y, Strauss S, et al. Parathyroid sonography: diagnostic accuracy related to shape, location, and texture of the gland. Br J Radiol 1987;60(713):439–43.

41. Lack EF, Clark MA, Buck DR, et al. Cysts of the para-thyroid gland: report of two cases and review of the literature. Am Surg 1978;44:376.

42. Krudy AG, Doppman JL, Shawker TH, et al. Hyper-functioning cystic parathyroid glands: computed tomography and sonographic findings. AJR Am J Roentgenol 1984;142:175.

43. Obara T, Fujimoto Y, Ito Y. Functioning parathyroid lipoadenoma-report of four cases: clinicopatholog-ical and ultrasonographic features. Endocrinol Jpn 1989;36:135.

44. American Institute of Ultrasound in Medicine. AIUM practice guideline for the performance of a thyroid and parathyroid ultrasound examination. J Ultra-sound Med 2003;22:1126–30.

45. Reeder SB, Desser TS, Weigel RJ, et al. Sonog-raphy in hyperparathyroidism: review with emphasis on scanning technique. J Ultrasound Med 2002;21:539.

46. Lane MJ, Desser TS, Weigel RJ, et al. Use of color and power Doppler sonography to identify feeding arteries associated with parathyroid adenomas. AJR Am J Roentgenol 1998;171:819.

47. Wolf RJ, Cronan JJ, Monchik JM. Color Doppler sonography: an adjunctive technique in assessment of parathyroid adenomas. J Ultrasound Med 1994;13:303.

48. Yeh MW, Barraclough BM, Sidhu SB, et al. Two hundred consecutive parathyroid ultrasound studies by a single clinician: the impact of experience. En-docr Pract 2006;12(3):257–63.

49. Doppman JL, Skarulis MC, Chen CC, et al. Parathy-roid adenomas in the aortopulmonary window. Radi-ology 1996;201(2):456–62.

50. Barraclough BM, Barraclough BH. Ultrasound of the thyroid and parathyroid glands. World J Surg 2000;24(2):158–65.

51. Huppert BJ, Reading CC. Parathyroid sonography: imaging and intervention. J Clin Ultrasound 2007;35(3):144–55.

52. Barbaros U, Erbil Y, Salmashoğlu A, et al. The char-acteristics of concomitant thyroid nodules cause false-positive ultrasonography results in primary hyperparathyroidism. Am J Otolaryngol 2009;30(4):239–43.

53. Ghaheri BA, Koslin DB, Wood AH, et al. Pre-operative ultrasound is worthwhile for reopera-tive parathyroid surgery. Laryngoscope 2004;114:2168–71.

54. Barczynski M, Golkowski F, Konturek A, et al. Tech-netium-99m-sestamibi subtraction scintigraphy vs. ultrasonography combined with a rapid parathyroid hormone assay in parathyroid aspirates in preopera-tive localization of parathyroid adenomas and in di-recting surgical approach. Clin Endocrinol (Oxf) 2006;65(1):106–13.

55. Heizmann O, Viehl CT, Schmid R, et al. Impact of concomitant thyroid pathology on preoperative workup for primary hyperparathyroidism. Eur J Med Res 2009;14(1):37–41.

56. Abboud B, Sleilaty G, Rabaa L, et al. Ultrasonog-raphy: highly accuracy technique for preoperative localization of parathyroid adenoma. Laryngoscope 2008;118(9):1574–8.

57. Mazzeo S, Caramella D, Lencioni R, et al. Useful-ness of echo-color Doppler in differentiating para-thyroid lesions from other cervical masses. Eur Radiol 1997;7(1):90–5.

58. Ahuja A, Ying M, King A, et al. Lymph node hilus: gray scale and power Doppler sonography of cervical nodes. J Ultrasound Med 2001;20: 987–92.

59. Solorzano CC, Carneiro-Pla DM, Irvin GL. Surgeon-performed ultrasonography as the initial and only localizing study in sporadic primary hyperparathyroidism. J Am Coll Surg 2006;202(1): 18–24.

60. Koslin DB, Adams J, Andersen P, et al. Preoperative evaluation of patients with primary hyperparathyroidism: role of high-resolution ultrasound. Laryngoscope 1997;107(9):1249–53.

61. Livingston CD, Victor B, Askew R, et al. Surgeon-performed ultrasonography as an adjunct to minimally invasive radio-guided parathyroidectomy in 100 consecutive patients with primary hyperparathyroidism. Endocr Pract 2008;14(1):28–32.

62. Stephen AE, Milas M, Garner CN, et al. Use of surgeon-performed office ultrasound and parathyroid fine needle aspiration for complex parathyroid localization. Surgery 2005;138(6):1143–50.

63. Veldman MW, Reading CC, Farrell MA, et al. Percutaneous parathyroid ethanol ablation in patients with multiple endocrine neoplasia type 1. AJR Am J Roentgenol 2008;191(6):1740–4.

Ultrasound-Guided Procedures for the Office

Russell B. Smith, MD[a,b,*]

KEYWORDS

- Ultrasound-guided • Fine-needle aspiration biopsy
- Interventional ultrasonography

⏵ Video versions of several figures in this article can be viewed at www.ultrasound.theclinics.com.

Over the past decade, ultrasonography (US) has become an instrumental component in the diagnostic evaluation of a multitude of head and neck pathologies. The technology can also be beneficial for image guidance during percutaneous and open head and neck procedures. Although US-guided fine-needle aspiration biopsy (FNAB) accounts for the vast majority of these procedures, US guidance can also be used for aspiration of fluid collections and therapeutic injections as well as an intraoperative adjuvant to guide revision surgery. A thorough understanding of the capabilities of interventional US allows optimal management of a wide variety of complex clinical scenarios.

FINE-NEEDLE ASPIRATION BIOPSY

Masses of the head and neck are frequently evaluated by FNAB to establish a diagnosis. Although some head and neck masses are easily palpable and hand-guided FNAB is feasible, many masses are indistinct or not palpable and image-guided FNAB is required. Additionally, it is not uncommon for a thyroid nodule or malignant adenopathy of the neck to be a complex mass with both solid and cystic components. In this situation, US guidance can decrease the chance of a nondiagnostic biopsy by ensuring that the solid component of the mass is sampled during the procedure. US-guided FNAB for nodular disease of the thyroid is the most commonly performed US-guided procedure, but salivary gland masses and cervical adenopathy as well as a wide variety of unusual neck masses may require image guidance for cytologic assessment. In addition to understanding the indications for biopsy and mastering the techniques of performing a US-guided biopsy, it is critical that otolaryngologists possess a thorough understanding of the limitations and potential pitfalls of FNAB in the assessment of masses in these areas.

Thyroid

In patients with thyroid nodules, many factors are considered when determining whether or not surgical intervention is required. Because most thyroid nodules are asymptomatic and nonfunctional, the key determinant of the need for surgery is the risk that a nodule represents a neoplasm. Although history, physical examination, and specific US features can assist otolaryngologists in determining the potential for neoplasm, FNAB is considered the most accurate diagnostic evaluation to assess for malignancy (Fig. 1). In patients with larger nodules, palpation-guided FNAB can be easily performed in the outpatient setting without the need for image guidance. But, many thyroid nodules are not easily palpable and image guidance is required to complete the biopsy. Additionally, some palpable thyroid nodules can be

This article was previously published in the December 2010 issue of *Otolaryngologic Clinics of North America*.
[a] Department of Otolaryngology—Head and Neck Surgery, 981225 University of Nebraska Medical Center, Omaha, NE 68198, USA
[b] Nebraska Methodist Estabrook Cancer Center, Omaha, NE, USA
* Department of Otolaryngology—Head and Neck Surgery, 981225 University of Nebraska Medical Center, Omaha, NE 68198.
E-mail address: rbsmith@unmc.edu

Ultrasound Clin 7 (2012) 219–228
doi:10.1016/j.cult.2011.12.006

A   B

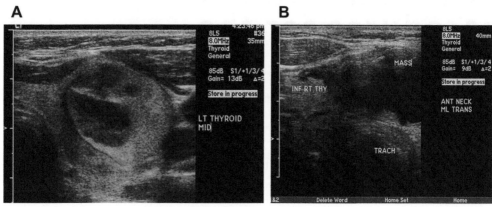

Fig. 1. US of thyroid nodules. Distinctly different-appearing thyroid nodules by US. (A) Thyroid nodule with US features suggestive of a benign nodule. (B) Thyroid nodule with US features suggestive of malignancy. Final histopathologic evaluation revealed both nodules to be follicular thyroid cancer.

complex masses with dominant cystic components. In this scenario, US guidance to ensure sampling of the solid component is valuable to ensure a diagnostic biopsy. Comparisons of palpation-guided and US-guided FNAB for thyroid nodules suggest that US-guided FNAB is more accurate and results in a lower rate of nondiagnostic biopsies. In a review of 376 FNABs of the thyroid, Izquierdo and colleagues[1] reported that for palpable thyroid nodules, US-guided FNAB was 20% more accurate (80%) and had a lower incidence of nondiagnostic specimens (7.1%) when compared with palpation-guided FNAB.

Recently, the National Cancer Institute proposed a 6-tiered classification scheme for the assessment of thyroid FNAB (Table 1).[2] Based on this system, the risk of malignancy for a thyroid nodule is defined and guidelines for management are proposed. In patients with nodules that by FNAB are suggestive of neoplasm, suspicious for malignancy, or malignant, surgery is recommended.[3] It is critical, however, to consider FNAB as only one component of the diagnostic evaluation of a patient with a thyroid nodule. In patients with history, physical examination, or imaging findings suggestive of malignancy, surgery should be recommended even if the FNAB is interpreted as low risk of malignancy.

In addition to the cytologic assessment of FNAB in a patient with suspected well-differentiated thyroid cancer, assessment for thyroglobulin in the saline washout of the needle after biopsy of a mass can be performed. Especially if a mass is suspected to be recurrent disease and has negative cytology, this technique can be a useful method to confirm the presence of disease. This technique can be used on masses suspected to be local or nodal recurrences, with the greatest benefit in lesions smaller than 1 cm.[4] After a 1-mL saline washout, a thyroglobulin of greater than 4 to 10 ng/mL has been established as indicative of disease, but false-positive results can occur.[4–6] This technique is valid even in patients who have antithyroglobulin antibodies.[7] Analysis for BRAF can also be completed on material obtained by FNAB in patients suspected of having

Table 1
National Cancer Institute thyroid FNAB guidelines committee IV

Suggested Category	Alternate Category	Risk of Malignancy
Benign		<1%
Atypia of undetermined significance	Indeterminant follicular lesions rule out neoplasm Atypical follicular lesion Cellular follicular lesion	5%–10%
Neoplasm	Suspicious for neoplasms	20%–30%
Suspicious for malignancy		50%–75%
Malignant		100%
Nondiagnostic	Unsatisfactory	—

papillary thyroid cancer. In the future, such an assessment may be important in surgical planning because patients with BRAF mutations are known to have more aggressive disease.[8]

In a fashion similar to thyroglobulin washout in patients with well-differentiated thyroid cancer, calcitonin washout can be performed in patients suspected of having primary or recurrent medullary thyroid cancer. In 36 patients suspected of having medullary thyroid cancer, the sensitivity and specificity of calcitonin washout has been reported as 100%, with FNAB cytologic evaluation having a sensitivity of 62% and specificity of 80%.[9] Although a calcitonin greater than 36 pg/mL is indicative of medullary thyroid cancer, others have found that patients with benign thyroid conditions can have calcitonin washout as high as 67 pg/mL and that in cases of medullary thyroid cancer the calcitonin washout was extremely high.[9,10]

Parathyroid

Unlike nodular disease of the thyroid, which routinely undergoes cytologic assessment, rarely is it necessary to perform FNAB for parathyroid pathology. For patients with hyperparathyroidism, the need for surgery is based on the metabolic sequelae of the disease rather than the concern that the disease represents malignancy. The success of parathyroidectomy for hyperparathyroidism is high with cure rates greater than 95%, obviating FNAB to confirm suspected lesions as parathyroid in origin.

In the small subset of patients who have persistent or recurrent hyperparathyroidism after prior surgical explorations, FNAB can play a role in the localization of the disease. In cases of persistent/recurrent disease, the pathology is usually located in the previously dissected central compartment. Subsequently, use of FNAB to confirm that suspicious lesions in previously operated fields are of parathyroid origin can be beneficial before revision surgery. When performing FNAB to confirm parathyroid disease, consider obtaining a parathyroid hormone washout of the aspirate in addition to cytologic assessment. Agrawal and colleagues reported limitations with cytologic evaluation of suspected parathyroid lesions by FNAB. In their series of 53 patients undergoing FNAB of suspected parathyroid lesions, the cytologic evaluation was able to identify parathyroid cells in only 40% of aspirates, with 28% of the aspirated being non-diagnostic.[11] Although the features of monomorphic cells with stippled nuclear chromatin in the absence of atypia, mitosis, or prominent nucleoli are suggestive of parathyroid origin, distinguishing parathyroid from thyroid tissue can be problematic especially if there is not any colloid in the specimen. Erbil and colleagues assessed the role of parathyroid hormone washout on the FNAB of lesions of the central compartment. Lesions suspected of parathyroid origin could be consistently discriminated from thyroid pathology with the parathyroid lesions having an average parathyroid hormone level of 4700 pg/mL compared to 48 pg/mL in the thyroid lesions.[12]

Salivary Gland

A wide variety of benign and malignant neoplasms can affect the major and minor salivary glands. Additionally, some non-neoplastic diseases can present as a salivary gland mass. The vast majority of salivary gland neoplasms are located in the parotid gland. The use of FNAB for salivary gland neoplasms is controversial, but it should be considered in the diagnostic evaluation of a patient with a salivary gland mass. Opponents of FNAB of salivary gland neoplasms feel that surgical excision should be performed for all tumors and that cytologic diagnosis does not significantly alter the treatment plan. Proponents of FNAB of salivary gland neoplasms feel that cytologic information assists in determining the risk of malignancy, allowing for optimal surgical planning and patient counseling preoperatively.

Given the wide variety of benign neoplasms as well as low-grade and high-grade malignancies that can affect the salivary glands, limitations exist regarding the ability of FNAB to establish a definitive diagnosis. Although some benign neoplasms, such as pleomorphic adenoma and Warthin tumor, can be accurately diagnosed by FNAB, other pathologies are more difficult to specifically classify on FNAB. For example, differentiating a cellular pleomorphic adenoma from a low-grade basal cell adenocarcinoma cannot be accomplished. Additionally, determining the exact pathologic subtype of a high-grade carcinoma is not possible (Table 2). The ability of US-guided FNAB of salivary gland neoplasms to distinguish benign from malignant tumors is high, with Bajaj and colleagues[13] reporting a sensitivity of 85%, specificity of 96%, and overall accuracy of 94%. Others have proposed core biopsy as the preferred technique for assessment of salivary gland neoplasms. Buckland and colleagues[14] reported 100% accuracy for US-guided core biopsy, with nearly all the masses in the series having undergone a prior FNAB that was nondiagnostic. The slightly more invasive nature of a core biopsy must be considered before implementing routine use of this technique. Overall, there is little doubt that FNAB can play a vital role in the assessment of select patients with a salivary gland mass.

Table 2
Erroneous diagnoses of fine-needle aspiration biopsy of salivary gland masses

Erroneous FNAB Result	Actual Diagnosis
Benign lymphoid tissue	Acinic cell carcinoma Lymphoma Warthin tumor
Non-neoplastic gland	Acinic cell carcinoma Pleomorphic adenoma Squamous cell carcinoma, mucoepidermoid carcinoma Warthin tumor
Pleomorphic adenoma	Adenoid cystic carcinoma
Basal cell adenoma	Basal cell adenocarcinoma Adenoid cystic carcinoma
Adenoid cystic carcinoma	Pleomorphic adenoma Basal cell adenoma

Lymph Node

Although a lateral neck mass may represent a wide variety of pathology, it is frequently the result of an enlarged lymph node. In patients with cervical lymphadenopathy, infectious, inflammatory, and neoplastic diagnoses must be considered. A patient's age, recent health status, history of exposure to carcinogens, and clinical characteristics of the mass are important factors in determining the probability that a neck mass may be malignant. FNAB is frequently performed on cervical lymphadenopathy to assess for malignancy before surgical excision of the mass. If possible, the surgeon should avoid the clinical scenario of performing an excisional biopsy of a lymph node and being surprised by the final pathology revealing carcinoma.

As with thyroid, parathyroid, and salivary gland pathology, US guidance for FNAB of cervical lymphadenopathy offers significant benefit. For malignant adenopathy, significant necrosis can be present and US guidance to the more solid areas of the lymph node can produce a higher yield of diagnostic biopsies. Conversely, in patients with presumed cervical lymphadenitis, US guidance can be used to access small areas of suppuration within the node to obtain a specimen for gram stain and cultures. Even in cases of suspected benign disease resulting in cervical lymphadenopathy, biopsy may play a role in establishing a diagnosis. Kim and colleagues reported on the use of US-guided core biopsies of cervical adenopathy in patients without known malignancy. Diagnostic specimens were obtained in 94% with a reported accuracy of 98% based on histologic confirmation of excisional biopsies or regression of suspected benign lesions.[15] The histologic diagnoses included reactive hyperplasia in 44 patients, tuberculosis in 37 patients, Kikuchi disease in 25 patients, metastasis in 16 patients, lymphoma in 16 patients, normal in 7 patients, and toxoplasmosis in 1 patient.

DRAINAGE PROCEDURES

Fluid collections are frequently encountered in the head and neck region. These collections may be the consequence of an infection with abscess formation, hemorrhage into an existing cyst, or a postoperative complication. US-guided drainage may be an appropriate intervention, depending on the clinical scenario, and allow an otolaryngologist to avoid an open surgical procedure for the management of the disease (**Fig. 2**). Chang and colleagues reported successful management of deep neck abscesses in 14 patients using US-guided drainage. Especially in patients with well-defined, unilocular abscesses, US drainage with or without drain placement should be considered without concern of complicating a future open drainage procedure if required.[16]

INJECTION PROCEDURES

Although injection procedures are the least commonly performed application of interventional US in the head and neck, it can be extremely valuable for certain clinical scenarios. These interventions may be for the injection of ablative or sclerosing agents or botulinum toxin A as well as placement of localization guide wires to assist with surgical resection (**Fig. 3**). Although these procedures can be safely performed, ensuring that the injection is not accidentally placed into a vascular structure is critical.

Success has been reported with the use of 95% ethanol for ablation of lesions in the head and neck, especially in those who are at high risk of undergoing surgical resection because of poor medical status or concerns of surgical morbidity due to prior therapy. This approach has been successfully performed for autonomous thyroid nodules, recurrent well-differentiated thyroid cancer, and recurrent primary hyperparathyroidism.[17–19] Some discomfort should be expected with these procedures and liberal application of local anesthetic in the skin as well as deeply around the area to be ablated should be performed. Temporary nerve paralysis has been reported with this technique.[19]

In patients with cerebral palsy, sialorrhea can be a major issue that negatively affects the quality of life of the patients as well as their caregivers.[20] Sialorrhea can also be a major issue in adults who

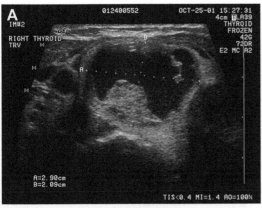
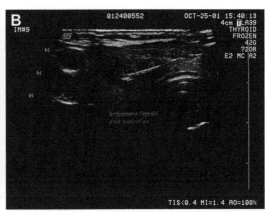

Fig. 2. US guidance for drainage of a thyroid hematoma. Patient presenting with an acutely enlarging mass in the thyroid. (*A*) US shows a complex-appearing mass with a large anechoic component. This was an intrathyroidal hematoma as a result of a neck trauma (strangulation). (*B*) US shows needle localized in area with near-total decompression of the hematoma. (*Courtesy of* Dr Robert Sofferman, MD.)

have degenerative neurologic diseases, such as Parkinson disease and amyotrophic lateral sclerosis.[21,22] For these conditions, intraglandular injection of botulinum toxin A can be effective in managing sialorrhea without a negative impact on the adjacent musculature. For these cases, US guidance to localize the needle within the parenchyma of the submandibular and the parotid glands can be used to ensure appropriate placement of the botulinum toxin A injection.

TECHNICAL CONSIDERATIONS IN INTERVENTIONAL ULTRASONOGRAPHY

To optimize the success of US-guided procedures, one must ensure that the patient is

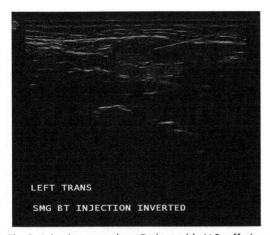

Fig. 3. Injection procedure. Patient with ALS suffering from sialorrhea. The US shows the needle with tip in submandibular gland. The hypoechoic changes noted at the tip of the needle is a result of the botulinum toxin A injection infiltrating the parenchyma of the gland. (*Courtesy of* Dr Lisa Orloff, MD.)

comfortably positioned and that the required supplies are available in the procedural suite. Developing a protocol/checklist for the staff assisting with the procedure can greatly facilitate this process. In addition to preparing the procedural room, the staff can assist with the procedure by manipulating the aspiration syringe as well as performing video documentation during the biopsy. Finally, communication with the Pathology department is critical to ensure that the biopsy specimen is prepared using methods that meet the needs of the cytologist.

Patient Preparation

Ensuring that the patient is comfortable for the procedure is critical to the success of US-guided interventions. If a patient is experiencing pain at the site of needle placement or is positioned such that the head and neck are not adequately supported, movement inevitably will occur. Any movement complicates needle placement and potentially decreases the success of the procedure.

Infiltration of the skin and subcutaneous tissues with local anesthetic should be completed before the procedure. An area approximately 2 cm in diameter should be anesthetized. The most efficient method to accurately place the local anesthetic is to put the patient in the identical position planned for the procedure. After positioning has been complete, US should be performed to localize the area of interest. Once the area of interest is well visualized with the probe positioned on the neck in the same fashion as it would be for the biopsy, the site at which the biopsy needle will enter the skin can be marked (**Fig. 4**). The local anesthetic can then be infiltrated around the area

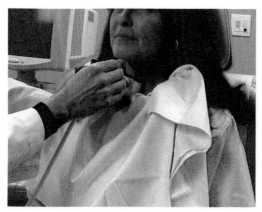

Fig. 4. Patient marking for local anesthetic infiltration. Once the US probe is localized in a position similar to that to be used for biopsy, the skin can be marked at the site at which the needle will be entered into the skin.

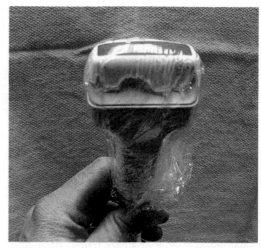

Fig. 5. Preparation of the US probe for needle biopsy. The US probe has US gel applied followed by coverage with a cling wrap before biopsy.

identified as the biopsy site. Additional local anesthetic can be placed along the planned needle path to the area to be biopsied if desired, but this is not frequently required.

Equipment and Supplies

As with diagnostic US of the head and neck, high-resolution US (8–12 MHz) should be used when performing image-guided procedures. Most commonly, a linear transducer is used during the procedure. It is important to optimize the setting of the US equipment based on the location and size of the mass to be biopsied. Ensure that the image contrast, magnification, and focal area are appropriately set before the procedure. The transducer must be prepared for the procedure to ensure that it is not exposed to body fluids or alcohol, which is used as asepsis for the skin. Several commercially available US probe covers are available, but cling wrap is a cost-effective alternative. A generous amount of US gel should be placed on the end of the transducer before placement of the protective barrier of choice (**Fig. 5**).

A multitude of supplies are required to perform percutaneous procedures in the head and neck (**Box 1**). Although alcohol preparation of the skin is adequate, Betadine or other sterile prep solutions can be considered per operator preference. Glass slides with fixative, Cytolye solution, and sterile containers for cultures should be prepared depending on the procedure being completed. Adhesive bandage and ice packs also need to be available for postprocedure care of the patient (**Fig. 6**).

The vast majority of FNAB are performed with either a 22Ga or a 25Ga needle. For drainage procedures, at least a 20Ga and preferably an 18Ga needle are used. The needle for injection procedures is typically a 25Ga needle, but if injecting a more viscous material, a larger needle may be required. A needle length of 1.5 in is adequate for the vast majority of lesions, but longer needles may be required for deep lesions or those that require a greater angle of approach to access the lesion. For fine-needle aspiration and drainage procedures, the needle may be directly attached to the syringe or an 8- to 12-in intravenous tubing may be used between the needle and the syringe. The advantage of using intravenous tubing is that it allows the assistant to manipulate the syringe for aspiration while the surgeon can focus efforts on

---

Box 1
Supplies for interventional ultrasonography

Alcohol prep pad

Skin marking pin

Syringe for local anesthetic

Syringe for aspiration

Needles (18, 22, 25, 27 Ga)

Local anesthetic

Intravenous tubing—optional

Needle aspiration gun—optional

Slides and fixative for smear preparation of the biopsy

CytoLyt for preparation of cell block

Adhesive bandage

Ice pack

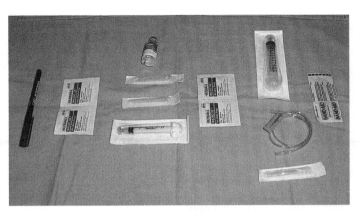

Fig. 6. Basic supplies used for office-based US procedures. Skin marker to mark site of local anesthetic infiltration; small syringe (3–5 μL) with needles for administration of local anesthetic; alcohol for skin prep before placement of anesthetic as well as biopsy; syringe and intravenous tubing; needle for biopsy; and adhesive bandage for biopsy site post procedure.

needle localization and movement within the area of interest depending on the procedure performed. For injection procedures, it is best to have the needle directly attached to the syringe to avoid waste of the injection material within the intravenous tubing.

Performing the Procedure

When performing US-guided procedures, two approaches can be used for needle placement. The approach used is predominantly influenced by the preference of the otolaryngologist performing the biopsy. In certain situations, one approach may be preferred due to anatomic considerations of the area of interest. The difference in the techniques is based on the relationship of the needle to the US transducer. The long-axis technique involves introducing the needle into the skin along the narrow side of transducer with the needle advanced parallel to area imaged (**Fig. 7**). With the short-axis technique, the needle is placed in the skin along the long side of the transducer and then advanced obliquely across the area imaged (**Fig. 8**).

Although the long-axis technique requires a slightly longer pathway to the area of interest, it has the advantage of allowing visualization of the entire needle during the procedure (**Fig. 9**). When using the long-axis technique, lesions that are deeply seated between anatomic structures may require that the US probe is oriented in the saggital plane instead of the axial plane when performing the biopsy. An example is a deeply located thyroid nodule positioned in between the trachea and carotid artery.

With the short-axis technique, a shorter needle pathway is used and almost every procedure can be performed while using axial imaging of the neck. The technique requires that the operator is comfortable seeing only the tip of the needle during the procedure instead of the entire needle (**Fig. 10**).

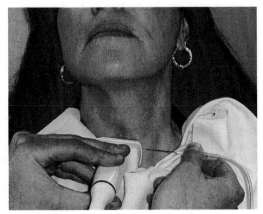

Fig. 7. Long-axis technique of needle placement. The needle is placed along the narrow side of transducer and advanced parallel to the imaged area.

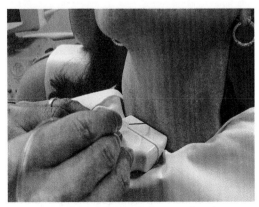

Fig. 8. Short-axis technique for needle placement. The needle is placed along the long side of transducer and advanced obliquely to the imaged area.

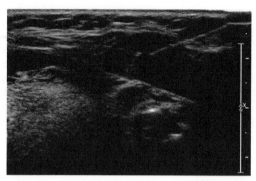

Fig. 9. US of long-axis technique. The entire needle path can be seen with the tip of the needle in the area to be biopsied. To see a video related to this figure please go to www.ultrasound.theclinics.com.

Considerations for Fine-Needle Aspiration Biopsy

Prior to inserting the needle into the area of interest, the plunger should be drawn back to allow at least 2 to 3 mL of air into the chamber. Once the needle is accurately placed into the mass of interest, slight negative pressure can be applied to the syringe and the needle is then moved rhythmically within the mass. Although sampling different areas of a mass should be considered, it is recommended that, with each biopsy, the needle passes focus on a small region and that each pass of the needle not randomly move to a different area of the mass.

With subsequent biopsies, a similar technique can be performed on different areas within the mass. The number of needle passes recommended varies and can be as few as 2 to 3 passes

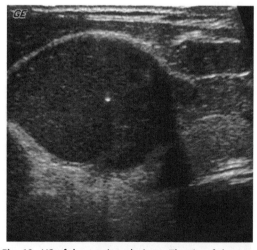

Fig. 10. US of short-axis technique. The tip of the needle is seen in the middle of the area of interest. To see a video related to this figure please go to www. ultrasound.theclinics.com.

and up to as many as 10 passes with each needle placement. Additional passes can be considered if no material is seen accumulating in the hub of the needle. Additionally, if a brisk return of blood or fluid is obtained, the number of needle passes in that area should be limited and the needle relocated to a different area of the mass. It must be ensured that the assistant has released all the negative pressure off the syringe before removing the needle from the area biopsied to avoid contaminants being drawn into the needle as well as to prevent the aspirate from being drawn all the way into the chamber of the syringe on exit of the skin.

Typically, three separate needle sampling are performed for each mass. Biopsy using a capillary technique has also been successful for cytologic assessment of a mass.[23] With this approach, a syringe is still needed to expel the biopsy material onto the slides once the biopsy has been completed.

Considerations for Drainage

A similar approach to FNAB may be used for drainage procedures. In this situation, the use of intravenous tubing has the advantages of allowing a surgeon to more freely move the needle to areas requiring drainage during the procedure while an assistant maintains negative pressure on the syringe. The use of intravenous tubing also allows the assistant to easily switch the syringe when filled so that the drainage procedure can be continued without having to remove the needle.

During the procedure, the surgeon should visualize the evacuation of the fluid collection. This allows the surgeon to move the needle to areas of residual fluid, which may be due to loculations or gravity-dependent areas in the neck. For larger fluid collections, external manipulation of the soft tissue of neck can be performed by the assistant to direct residual fluid toward the needle to facilitate evacuation of the area. Percutaneous drain placement can be considered as part of the procedure based on the management requirements of the disease.

Injection

Injection of therapeutic agents using US guidance ensures delivery of the agent to the target area and not into adjacent critical structures. For most procedures, a volume of less than 1 mL is used. Injection of small volumes helps ensure that limited to no extravasation of the injected agent occurs. For botulinum toxin A injections, each gland receives two intraglandular injections with a total dose of 125 U required.[21] For ethanol ablative therapy, a total volume of 0.5 to 1 mL is injected as multiple 0.1-mL aliquots throughout the mass. With ethanol therapy, the area injected quickly becomes intensely echogenic. This lasts approximately 1 minute and should be allowed to resolve before attempting additional injections to ensure that the needle tip is not obscured.[18,19] Other agents may also be used depending on the clinical scenario and the specific characteristics of each agent must be understood to allow safe injection.

CONCLUSION: APPLICATIONS FOR INTERVENTIONAL ULTRASOUND OF HEAD AND NECK

There are many applications for interventional US in the head and neck. Although FNAB is the most common performed image-guided procedure, a host of other interventions can be of clinical benefit. The success of US-guided procedures is dependent on many factors, but the technique can be easily mastered by otolaryngologists.

REFERENCES

1. Izquierdo R, Arekat MR, Knudson PE, et al. Comparison of palpation-guided and ultrasound-guided fine-needle biopsies of thyroid nodules in an outpatient endocrinology practice. Endocr Pract 2006;12:609–14.
2. Baloch ZW, Ciabs ES, Clak DP, et al. The National Cancer Institute thyroid fine needle aspiration state of the science conference: a summation. Cytojournal 2008;5:6.
3. Layfield LJ, Cibas ES, Gharib H, et al. Thyroid aspiration cytology: current status. CA Cancer J Clin 2009;59:99–110.
4. Lee YH, Seo HS, Suh SI, et al. Cut-off value for needle washout thyroglobulin in athyrotropic patients. Laryngoscope 2010;120:1120–4.
5. Mikosiriski S, Pomorski L, Oszukowska L, et al. The diagnostic value of thyroglobulin concentration in fine-needle aspiration of the cervical lymph nodes in patients with differentiated thyroid cancer. Endorkrynol Pol 2006;57:392–5.
6. Kim MJ, Kim EK, Kim BM, et al. Thyroglobulin measurement in fine-needle aspiration washouts: the criteria for neck node dissection for patients with thyroid cancer. Clin Endocrinol (Oxf) 2009;70:145–51.
7. Boi F, Baghino G, Atzeni F, et al. The diagnostic value for differentiated thyroid carcinoma metastases of thyroglobulin (Tg) measurement in washout fluid from fine-needle aspiration biopsy of neck lymph nodes is maintained in the presence of circulating anti-Tg antibodies. J Clin Endocrinol Metab 2006;91:1364–9.
8. Xing M. BRAF mutation in thyroid cancer. Endocr Relat Cancer 2005;12:245–62.
9. Boi F, Maurelli I, Pinna G, et al. Calcitonin measurement in wash-out fluid from fine needle aspiration of neck masses in patients with primary and metastatic medullary thyroid carcinoma. Clin Endocrinol Metab 2007;92:2115–8.
10. Kudo T, Miyauchi A, Ito Y, et al. Diagnosis of medullary thyroid carcinoma by calcitonin measurement in fine-needle aspiration biopsy specimens. Thyroid 2007;17:635–8.
11. Agarwal AM, Bentz JS, Hungerford R, et al. Parathyroid fine-needle aspiration cytology in the evaluation of parathyroid adenoma: cytologic findings from 53 patients. Diagn Cytopathol 2009;37:407–10.
12. Erbil Y, Barbaros U, Salmaslioglu A, et al. Value o13.f parathyroid hormone assay for preoperative sonographically guided parathyroid aspirates for minimally invasive parathyroidectomy. J Clin Ultrasound 2006;34:425–9.
13. Bajaj Y, Singh S, Cozens N, et al. Critical clinical appraisal of the role of ultrasound guided fine needle aspiration cytology in the management of parotid tumors. J Laryngol Otol 2005;119:289–92.
14. Buckland JR, Manjaly G, Violaris N, et al. Ultrasound-guided cutting needle biopsy of the parotid gland. J Laryngol Otol 1999;113:988–92.
15. Kim BM, Kim EK, Kim MJ, et al. Sonographically guided core needle biopsy of cervical lymphadenopathy in patients without known malignancy. J Ultrasound Med 2007;26:585–91.
16. Chang KP, Chen YL, Hao SP, et al. Ultrasound-guided closed drainage for abscesses of the head and neck. Otolaryngol Head Neck Surg 2005;132:119–24.
17. Golletti O, Monzani F, Caraccio N, et al. Percutaneous ethanol injection treatment of autonomously functioning single thyroid nodules: optimization of treatment and short term outcome. World J Surg 1992;16:784–9.
18. Lewis BD, Hay ID, Charboneau JW, et al. Percutaneous ethanol injection for treatment of cervical lymph node metastases in patients with papillary thyroid carcinoma. Am J Roentgenol 2002;178:699–704.
19. Harman CR, Grant CS, Hay ID, et al. Indications, technique, and efficacy of alcohol injection of enlarged parathyroid glands in patients with primary hyperparathyroidism. Surgery 1998;124:1011–20.
20. Banerjee KJ, Glasson C, O'Flaherty SJ. Parotid and submandibular botulinum toxin A injections for sialorrhea in children with cerebral palsy. Dev Med Child Neurol 2006;48:883–7.
21. Nobrega AC, Rodrigues B, Melo A. Does botulinum toxin injection in parotid glands interfere with the swallowing dynamics of Parkinson's disease patients? Clin Neurol Neurosurg 2009;111:430–2.

22. Gilio F, Iacovelli E, Frasca V, et al. Botulinum toxin type A for treatment of sialorrhea in amyotropic lateral sclerosis: a clinical and neurophysiologic study. Amyotroph Lateral Scler 2010;11:359–63.

23. De Carvalho GA, Paz-Filho G, Cavalcanti TC, et al. Adequacy and diagnostic accuracy of aspiration vs. capillary fine needle thyroid biopsies. Endocr Pathol 2009;20:204–8.

Head and Neck Ultrasound in the Pediatric Population

Veronica J. Rooks, MD[a,b], Benjamin B. Cable, MD[a,c],*

KEYWORDS
- Pediatric • Head and neck ultrasound • Otolaryngology
- Office imaging

ADVANTAGES OF OFFICE IMAGING STUDIES OF THE HEAD AND NECK IN CHILDREN

Diagnostic imaging studies of the head and neck in children have three main challenges. First, pediatric conditions that require imaging are often dynamic and changing. Examples include lymphadenopathy, deep neck space infections, and vascular malformations. Although an initial imaging study can offer a great deal of information, it remains a snapshot in time and does not offer the physician insight beyond a narrow period. Many pediatric lesions quickly evolve over days or weeks, making remote imaging less relevant. Also, virtually all pediatric imaging is done outside the otolaryngology clinic. This not only requires additional logistics but also is accompanied by an interruption in care. In most major medical centers, imaging is scheduled hours, days, or weeks after the initial clinic visit. Once completed, the study must be conveyed back to the managing provider for review and decision making. Finally, many pediatric imaging studies require sedation or even general anesthesia for adequate information to be gained. This adds further logistical challenges to the health care team and poses additional risk to the patient.

In selected cases, directed ultrasound has the potential to solve all three of these major issues.

Ultrasound devices are now portable enough to be brought directly to the operating room, clinic examination room, or bedside and can be used by a radiologist or otolaryngologist with little preparation. Examinations are usually completed in minutes, can frequently be performed during the initial consultation, and are well tolerated in most children. With no need for radiation exposure, intravenous medication, or sedation, it can be repeated as often as needed rather than offering a single snap-shot of the lesion in question; ultrasound can be repeatedly used to track the evolution of lesions before, sometimes during, and after treatment.

Pediatric head and neck ultrasound uses the same hardware used in adult applications. No additional supplies are needed. Machines range in size from moderate-sized carts to laptop versions that are placed on wheeled stands. Each of the machines fit into a standard size examination room and, with battery backup, can be moved between treatment areas without interruption. Image storage varies between machines and ranges across the standard data formats and, depending on hospital archive systems, may or may not be available throughout the hospital. Although many probe types exist, a single high-frequency linear probe, 8 to 15 MHz, is adequate for most applications in otolaryngology.

This article was previously published in the December 2010 issue of *Otolaryngologic Clinics of North America*.
The authors have no financial disclosures.
a Uniformed Services University of the Health Sciences, Bethesda, MD, USA
b Pediatric Radiology, Department of Radiology, Tripler Army Medical Center, 1 Jarrett White Road, TAMC, Honolulu, HI 96859, USA
c Pediatric Otolaryngology/Head & Neck Surgery, Tripler Army Medical Center, 3C ENT Clinic, 1 Jarrett White Road, Honolulu, TAMC, HI 96859, USA
* Corresponding author. Pediatric Otolaryngology/Head & Neck Surgery, Tripler Army Medical Center, 3C ENT Clinic, 1 Jarrett White Road, Honolulu, TAMC, HI 96859.
E-mail address: benjamin.cable@us.army.mil

Ultrasound Clin 7 (2012) 229–237
doi:10.1016/j.cult.2011.12.007

Specific courses in pediatric ultrasound for otolaryngologists do not yet exist. Despite this lack, current course offerings dealing with adult ultrasound are offered to otolaryngologists through the American College of Surgeons. Techniques reviewed and evaluated at these training events are highly relevant to pediatric applications. Along with outside training, partnership with one's own radiology team is indispensable for advice and training as comfort is gained with the basic examination and techniques.

SPECIFIC APPLICATIONS OF ULTRASOUND IN THE OTOLARNGOLOGY CLINIC
Lymphadenopathy

Evaluation of lymphadenopathy in children can quickly be accomplished with ultrasound. In the authors' clinic, ultrasound has evolved to become a natural extension of the physical examination. Although palpation of lymphadenopathy in most children is simple, accurate sizing of lymph nodes and diagnosis of multiple contiguous nodes is often

difficult. Overlying tissue frequently adds to the perceived size of the lymph nodes. Ultrasound offers solutions to both problems. With a brief imaging examination done to enhance palpation, the location of the lymphadenopathy is quickly determined. Precise sizing can be performed with digital calipers. Specific nodal architecture can often be visualized. Normal or reactive lymph nodes should typically be well defined and elliptical in shape. Their parenchyma should be homogeneously hypoechoic with a central linear-hyperechoic vascular hilum (**Fig. 1**). Although no ultrasound findings have been strongly correlated with neoplasm, concerns for malignancy arise with loss of the normal architecture, loss of the kidney bean shape to a more bulbous or round shape, absent hilum, irregular borders, cystic necrosis, and irregular capsular vasculature.[1] With baseline data established during initial consultation, children can be monitored with serial ultrasound examinations while undergoing medical evaluation and treatment. Any nodes that remain enlarged or demonstrate multiple abnormal

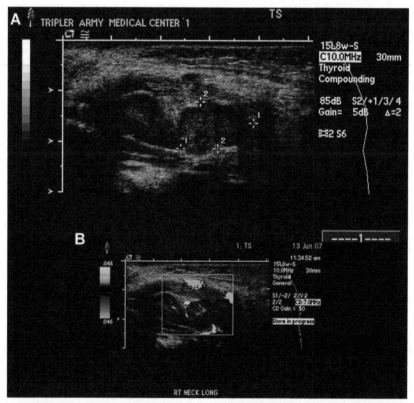

Fig. 1. (A) Five-month-old with fevers to 103°F for 36 hours with increased swelling of right neck. Screening ultrasound images demonstrate bilobed solid structures with hypoechoic peripheral parenchyma and central increased hilar echogenicity, consistent with a reactive lymph node. (B) Central color Doppler flow is noted, characteristic for a lymph node. Electronic calipers allow incremental follow-up to the scale of a millimeter.

findings despite treatment can be documented and targeted for excisional biopsy as indicated.

Branchial Cleft Anomalies and Thyroglossal Duct Cysts

Ultrasound can be used to evaluate branchial cleft anomalies and thyroglossal duct cysts (**Figs. 2 and 3**). In each case, cysts often present as thin-walled ovoid or round masses with significant heterogeneity and a lack of vascular architecture. Because 90% of branchial cleft cysts have origins in the second arch, most are frequently confirmed to be anterior to the sternocleidomastoid whereas thyroglossal duct cysts are most frequently localized within or in close proximity to the strap musculature.[2] Thyroglossal duct cysts can, in rare circumstances, represent ectopic thyroid tissue.

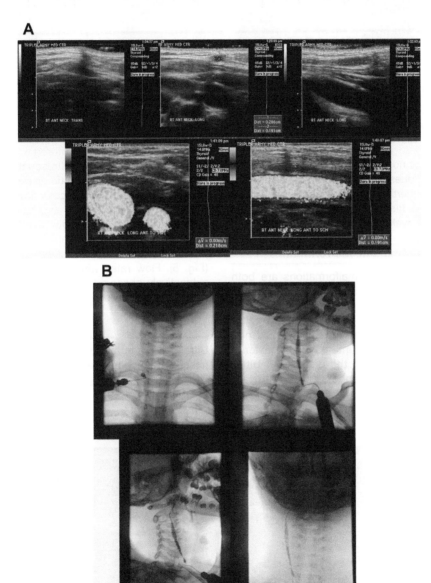

Fig. 2. (*A*) Five-year-old's complaint of "orange juice comes out this hole in my neck." Thyroglossal duct fistula ultrasound images demonstrate transverse and longitudinal images of the hypoechoic tract extending from skin surface, heading superiorly along carotid artery. (*B*) Fluoroscopic spot images after catheritization with angiocatheter and injection of contrast media demonstrate fistula tract from skin surface to pyriform sinus, consistent with branchial cleft fistula. (*C*) Axial and coronal reformatted images demonstrate skin orifice origin at the inferior-middle two-thirds junction of sternocleidomastoid muscle (SCM); deep to platysma; lateral to cranial nerves IX, X, and XII; between the internal and external carotid; and terminating in the tonsillar fossa.

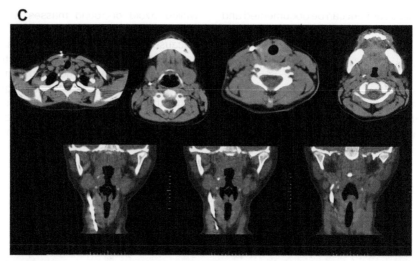

Fig. 2. (*continued*)

Confirmation of normal thyroid architecture below the mass in question is recommended before surgery is undertaken.[3] Ultrasound can easily accomplish this task during the same examination done for mass evaluation.

Vascular and Lymphatic Malformations

Vascular and lymphatic malformations are both amenable to ultrasound evaluation. Although various classification schemes exist, mixed lesions are possible and, in the authors' opinion, more frequent than often reported. Purely lymphatic malformations are often encountered in the posterior cervical space and within the oral cavity. Ultrasound examination demonstrates cysts with variable thickness to their septa and heterogeneous

fluid levels within (**Fig. 4**).[2] Ultrasound examination can rapidly define microcystic disease from macrocystic elements. Doppler color flow examination is invaluable in this setting and quickly confirms lack of significant blood flow. Finding significant random blood flow patterns within a lesion provides evidence for a vascular or mixed lesion (**Fig. 5**). Flow rates within these lesions can be subjectively observed and low-flow versus high-flow status can be seen in real time.

Abscesses

Ultrasound can be used to evaluate possible abscess formation. Classically, deep neck space infections have been limited to expansion within potential spaces and limited by fascial planes.

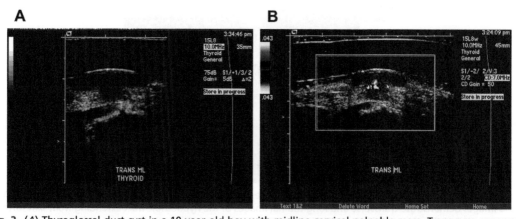

Fig. 3. (*A*) Thyroglossal duct cyst in a 10-year-old boy with midline cervical palpable mass. Transverse sonogram demonstrates an oval, well-defined, hypoechoic mass with through transmission in the suprahyoid neck midline. Note anechoic standoff pad placed between transducer and skin surface to facilitate superficial lesions. (*B*) Color Doppler imaging demonstrates peripheral color Doppler flow without central flow. Echogenic debris centrally with lack of color flow is consistent with a cystic structure with central sloughed cells.

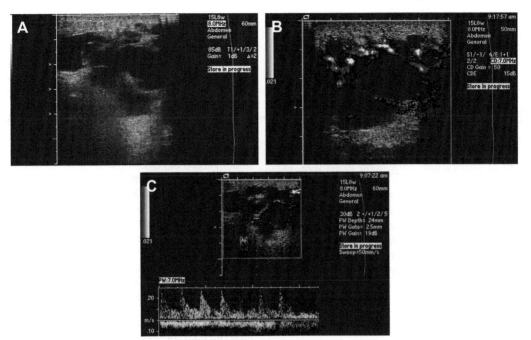

Fig. 4. (A) Three-year-old girl with palpable neck mass demonstrating thin-walled, multicystic masses with septae of variable thickness. Echogenic fluid may simulate solid lymph node or fluid-fluid levels may demonstrate area of recent hemorrhage into the cystic cavity. (B) Color power Doppler imaging demonstrates flow within the septae with (C) depicting an arterial waveform within septations.

With the advent of methicillin-resistant *Staphylococcus aureus*, otolaryngologists have begun to see more cases of superficial cellulitis lead to abscesss formation.[4,5] These superficial abscesses with overlying cellulitis are often difficult to examine by palpation alone. Ultrasound again offers an augmentation of the physical examination in these situations and can quickly identify

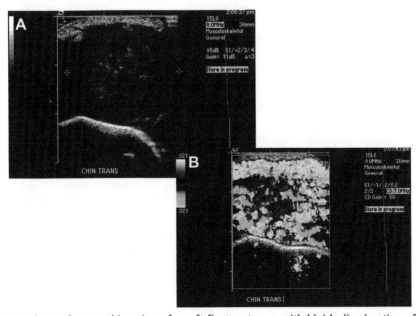

Fig. 5. (A) Hemangioma ultrasound imaging of a soft fluctuant mass with bluish discoloration of chin present since birth. Gray scale demonstrates slightly heterogenous hypoechogenicity with (B) intense diffuse color Doppler flow of the highly vascularized channels lines by endothelial cells, characteristic for hemangioma.

the border between soft tissue and the pus within an abscess cavity. Needle localization with or without excision and drainage can follow and total evacuation of the cavity can be confirmed.

Other Applications

Many other clinical applications for diagnostic ultrasound have been reported in the pediatric population. Infants born with an anterior neck mass and torticollis can be evaluated for pseudo-tumor of infancy with ultrasound alone (**Fig. 6**).[6] This modality can be used in the clinic to obviate CT or MRI evaluation. Laryngeal studies in children have been undertaken to assess dynamic vocal cord function and papilloma status in patients with known disease.[7,8] Thyroid mass evaluation can be performed in children as it is done in adults. Finally, ultrasonography has even been found to be an accurate method of confirming middle ear fluid and further defining the viscosity of the effusion.[9]

SPECIFIC APPLICATIONS IN THE OTOLARYNGOLOGY OPERATING ROOM
Intralesional Laser Treatment of Vascular Lesions

First introduced to the pediatric otolaryngology community by Brietzke and colleagues in 2001, intralesional laser treatment has become a viable tool for treating the spectrum of vascular lesions.[10] Using this technique, ultrasound evaluation is performed in a clinical setting and then confirmed at the time of surgery. Under ultrasound guidance, an 18-gauge intravenous catheter is introduced into the lesion and directed toward small to medium-sized feeding vasculature or central parenchyma (**Fig. 7**). Using a 600-μm fiber introduced through the intravenous catheter, a neody-mium:yttrium-aluminum-garnet laser is delivered using 6 to 10 W of power using a continuous mode (**Fig. 8**). Color Doppler flow can be used to track the effect of the laser energy in real time. As the laser is applied over a 5- to 20-second span, the coagulative effect is visible expanding from a few millimeters to 1.5 cm from the tip of the fiber. Using this technique, the lesion can be coagulated by region or vessel. Direct results are visible as the Doppler flow detected decreases and echogenicity of the surrounding tissue increases. Care must be taken to avoid any significant heating of the overlying skin or mucosa because bleeding and tissue loss are both possible. Great care must also be taken with higher flow lesions because air may be draw into catheters if left open and air embolus may result. Intralesional therapy can also be used as part of a multimodality approach to disease (**Fig. 9**).

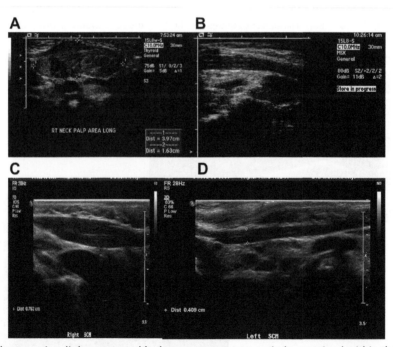

Fig. 6. Initial fibromatosis coli demonstrated by heterogenous mass entirely contained within the right SCM (*A*) with contralateral normal left SCM (*B*). Two month follow-up after physical therapy demonstrates interval improvement on the heterogenous mass (*C*) with only slight increased thickness remaining in comparison to the normal left SCM (*D*).

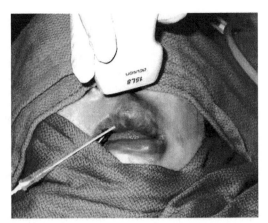

Fig. 7. A 600-μm fiber introduced via an 18-gauge angiocatheter. Tape is used to mark appropriate depth of fiber within catheter.

Fine-Needle and Core Needle Biopsy

Fine-needle aspiration (FNA) has become a mainstay in the initial evaluation of adult lymphadenopathy. Although the pediatric malignancy spectrum makes the need for FNA less common, there are still several situations where an FNA or a core needle biopsy would be of value. Examples include enlarged parotid nodes where an excisional biopsy is difficult and any situation where direct excision is contraindicated. Although most children require the addition of sedation or anesthesia to tolerate skin penetration, ultrasound-guided biopsy offers the same advantages in children as it does in adults. Direct nodal penetration can be observed and tissue can be removed from areas throughout the node (**Fig. 10**). Needle penetration is controlled and deep structures can be preserved from needle trauma. If nodal architecture is required, core needle specimens can be taken.

Localization of Botulinum Toxin Injections for Sialorrhea and Spastic Muscular Pathology

Socially disruptive sialorrhea is a common problem encountered by children with neurologic disease. Gland removal, duct rerouting, and duct ligations are all possible options but each technique is irreversible and destructive. Botox injection into the submandibular and parotid glands is a treatment that offers the patient and family

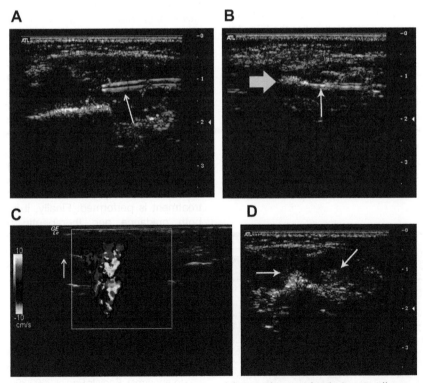

Fig. 8. (*A*) Catheter (*arrow*) visible within center of lesion. (*B*) Firing laser within lesion. Small arrow denotes 600-μm fiber protruding from catheter. Large arrow denotes increasing echogenicity of tissue as coagulation occurs. (*C*) Fiber introduced via catheter from left (*small arrow*). Color Doppler flow represents laser energy emanating from tip of fiber superiorly, artifact inferiorly. (*D*) Lesion after laser treatment. Arrows denote significant increase in echogenicity of treated areas.

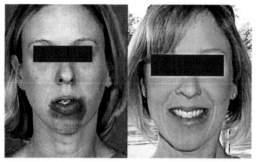

Fig. 9. Patient before and after multimodality treatment of vascular lesion. Patient underwent intralesional and pulsed dye laser treatment followed by a single debulking of the left lateral lower lip.

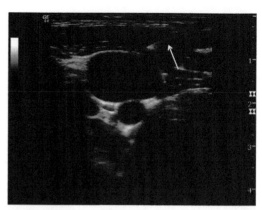

Fig. 11. Needle placed within spastic SCM muscle. Note close proximity to vasculature (*arrow*).

a nondestructive and temporary solution. In this way, a family is able to evaluate or trial the effects of the more permanent procedures. Ultrasound is an invaluable tool for the guidance of Botox injection, which is usually done in an operating room under anesthesia. Using ultrasound localization, Botox can be directly injected into multiple areas of each gland while taking care to avoid extravasation of toxin to surrounding musculature. Identical procedures can be used to localize Botox to spastic muscle groups in the neck when treating patients for otherwise intractable disease (**Fig. 11**).

Other Potential Applications

Although many methods of airway control are familiar to pediatric otolaryngologists, ultrasound confirmation of endotracheal tube placement has been described and offers an additional potential tool.[11] Intraoperative ultrasound localization of deep neck space abscesses has been described as an adjunctive method for incision and drainage procedures.[12] Finally, minimally invasive tongue

base reduction surgery has been described, in which ultrasound is used to map both lingual arteries while submucosal tissue is removed from between each.[13]

ULTRASOUND AS A TOOL FOR THE OTOLARYNGOLOGIST

Ultrasound, as a diagnostic modality, has been developing rapidly. High-resolution ultrasound machines have now been reduced to the size of a laptop computer. In years past, ultrasound use was largely limited to radiology departments but this is changing. Ultrasound can be easily adopted by otolaryngologists for use within the clinic and the operating room. Keys to adoption include training and close partnerships with radiology colleagues. Ultrasound seems to offer several particular advantages to the pediatric patient population. It is well tolerated and quickly adds a degree of precision to the physical examination. It can be done repeatedly as lesions evolve and treatment is performed. Finally, it is valuable for both guidance and therapeutic treatment of lesions in the operating room. With each of these benefits, it is likely that ultrasound use will continue to rapidly grow and evolve as a tool within the field of otolaryngology.

REFERENCES

1. Restrepo R, Oneto J, Lopez K, et al. Head and neck lymph nodes in children: the spectrum from normal to abnormal. Pediatr Radiol 2009;39(8):836–46.
2. Meuwly JY, Lepori D, Theumann N, et al. Multimodality imaging evaluation of the pediatric neck: techniques and spectrum of findings. Radiographics 2005;25(4):931–48.

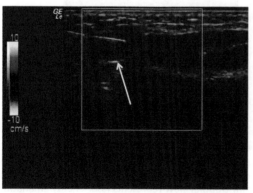

Fig. 10. Needle precisely placed within lymph node (*arrow*).

3. Gupta P, Maddalozzo J. Preoperative sonography in presumed thyroglossal duct cysts. Arch Otolaryngol Head Neck Surg 2001;127(2):200–2.

4. Bothwell NE, Shvidler J, Cable BB. Acute rise in methicillin-resistant Staphylococcus aureus infections in a coastal community. Otolaryngol Head Neck Surg 2007;137(6):942–6.

5. Inman JC, Rowe M, Ghostine M, et al. Pediatric neck abscesses: changing organisms and empiric therapies. Laryngoscope 2008;118(12):2111–4.

6. Maddalozzo J, Goldenberg JD. Pseudotumor of infancy—the role of ultrasonography. Ear Nose Throat J 1996;75(4):248–54.

7. Friedman EM. Role of ultrasound in the assessment of vocal cord function in infants and children. Ann Otol Rhinol Laryngol 1997;106(3):199–209.

8. Bryson PC, Leight WD, Zdanski CJ, et al. High-resolution ultrasound in the evaluation of pediatric recurrent respiratory papillomatosis. Arch Otolaryngol Head Neck Surg 2009;135(3):250–3.

9. Discolo CM, Byrd MC, Bates T, et al. Ultrasonic detection of middle ear effusion: a preliminary study. Arch Otolaryngol Head Neck Surg 2004;130(12): 1407–10.

10. Brietzke S, Therberge D, Mair E. Nd:YAG interstitial laser therapy for pediatric arteriovenous malformations. Operat Tech Otolaryngol Head Neck Surg 2001;12(4):239–44.

11. Galicinao J, Bush AJ, Godambe SA. Use of bedside ultrasonography for endotracheal tube placement in pediatric patients: a feasibility study. Pediatrics 2007;120(6):1297–303.

12. Duque CS, Guerra L, Roy S. Use of intraoperative ultrasound for localizing difficult parapharyngeal space abscesses in children. Int J Pediatr Otorhinolaryngol 2007;71(3):375–8.

13. Maturo SC, Mair EA. Submucosal minimally invasive lingual excision: an effective, novel surgery for pediatric tongue base reduction. Ann Otol Rhinol Laryngol 2006;115(8):624–30.

Emerging Technology in Head and Neck Ultrasonography

Michael R. Holtel, MD[a,b,*]

KEYWORDS

- Ultrasound technology • Microbubbles
- Ultrasound hemostasis • Head and neck ultrasound
- Elastography

ULTRASOUND: CURRENT AND FUTURE USE

Ultrasonography of the head and neck is currently a cost-effective imaging tool allowing assessment beyond the clinician's physical examination. Ultrasonography is uniquely portable when compared with other imaging modalities, making it ideal for use in the clinical setting. It provides the clinician immediate feedback, allowing the provider to make accurate assessments in a timely manner. Ultrasonography does not carry the risk of irradiation and has been the tool of choice for diagnostic and therapeutic interventions, such as fine-needle aspiration and line placement.

Ultrasound technology has distinct advantages in these areas, with continued advances and new technology likely to emerge. To allow increased ease of use in the clinical settling, palm-sized ultrasound machines are being produced, which are likely to be miniaturized even further. The ability to palpate with the ultrasound probe provides unique information on a lesion's compressibility or stiffness not available with computerized tomography (CT) and magnetic resonance imaging (MRI). This "objective" palpation is proving useful in determining whether a lesion is benign or malignant. Although attempts to use ultrasonography for therapeutic intervention in the head and neck date back to its use in Ménière disease in 1960,[1] it is in therapeutic intervention that future applications show the most promise. Two promising therapeutic ultrasound interventions are the use of (1) drug-containing *microbubbles* that, using ultrasound, can release an antitumor agent, deliver gene therapy, or release other therapeutic substances at the target tissue and (2) focused ultrasound to coagulate bleeding vessels or destroy inaccessible tumors.

Discussions on emerging technology in ultrasonography in this article are limited to those in which there is clinical evidence to support the benefit, although in some cases that evidence is not specific to the head and neck.

MACHINE SIZE

Laptop ultrasound systems are increasingly common. Several manufacturers are introducing palm-sized ultrasound machines, including the Acuson P10 (Siemens Medical Solutions Inc, Malvern, PA, USA) introduced in 2007, the Signos (Signostics Inc, Palo Alto, CA, USA) introduced in 2009, and the Vscan (GE Healthcare, Piscataway, NJ, USA) in 2010. Although the palm-sized machines are currently designed for vascular access, bladder examination, and trauma settings, it is likely that they will eventually be improved to provide the image quality necessary for use in head and neck examination (**Fig. 1**).

This article was previously published in the December 2010 issue of *Otolaryngologic Clinics of North America*. The views expressed are those of the author and do not represent the views of the US Army, US military, Sharp Rees Stealy Medical Group or the University of Hawaii.

[a] Telemedicine Research Institute, University of Hawaii, 651 Ilalo Street, Honolulu, HI 96813, USA
[b] Telemedicine and Advanced Technology Research Center of the United States Army Medical Readiness and Materiel Command, MCMR-TT (TATRC) Building 1054 Patchel Street, Ft Detrick, MD 21702-5012, USA
* Sharp Rees Stealy Medical Group, 10670 Wexford Street, San Diego, CA 92131.
E-mail address: mholtel@gmail.com

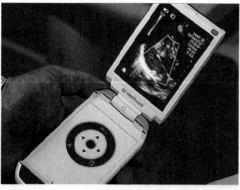

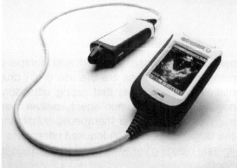

Fig. 1. Palm-sized ultrasound machines. (*Courtesy of* Signotics Inc, USA [Web site: superdupertech.com/2009/05]; with permission.)

PALPATION WITH ELASTOGRAPHY

Ultrasound examiners have long used palpation of masses with the ultrasound probe as an adjunct to their visual examination. Ultrasound elastography provides a more objective measurement of stiffness or, in more precise physics terms, strain. Changes in returning echoes are measured at the transducer before being converted to B-mode ultrasound before and after compression with the ultrasound transducer. The difference is depicted on an elastogram as lighter for less dense and darker for more dense tissue or masses (**Figs. 2** and **3**). Since its approval by US Food and Drug Administration in 2006, ultrasound elastography has been used to discriminate between malignant and benign breast masses based on its objective measure of the stiffness of those masses. There is initial evidence that ultrasound elastography may be useful in differentiating between benign and malignant thyroid nodules. Scoring tissue stiffness on ultrasound elastography from 1 (low stiffness) to 6 (high stiffness), Hong and colleagues[2] in 2009 demonstrated in 90 consecutive surgical patients that 86 of 96 benign thyroid nodules (90%) had a score of 1 to 3, whereas 43 of 49 malignant thyroid nodules (88%) had a score of

4 to 6. Similarly, Rago and colleagues[3] in 2007 used a scoring from 1 to 5 based on elastography in 92 consecutive patients undergoing thyroidectomy for compressive symptoms or suspicion of malignancy. Low stiffness scores of 1 and 2 were found in 49 cases, all benign thyroid nodules; scores of 3, in 13 cases, one malignant and 12 benign thyroid lesions; and high stiffness scores of 4 and 5, in 30 cases, all carcinomas. Sensitivity in these 2 studies ranged from 88% to 90% and specificity, from 90% to 100%. Asteria and colleagues[4] in 2008 in a third study of 67 patients with 86 thyroid nodules used stiffness scores of 1 through 4 and found slightly higher specificity for malignancy of 94%, but a decreased sensitivity of 81%. There remains some doubt over interobserver reliability of ultrasound elastography for the thyroid nodule.

REPLACING PALPATION WITH SOUND USING SONOELASTOGRAPHY AND ACOUSTIC RADIATION FORCE IMAGING

In place of manual palpation (displacement) with the transducer, sonoelastography uses Doppler ultrasound to detect movement in a neck mass created by an external vibration. Lyshchik and colleagues[5] in 2007 examined 141 cervical lymph nodes in 43 patients with suspected hypopharyngeal or thyroid cancer using ultrasound sonoelastography. Stiffness or strain of the lymph node and surrounding muscle was measured. When the ratio of muscle/lymph node strain was greater than 1.5, they found a 98% specificity, 85% sensitivity, and 92% overall accuracy of identifying metastatic lymph nodes. Dighe and colleagues[6] used compression generated by the carotid artery on thyroid masses along with Doppler ultrasound to determine stiffness or strain in 53 patients with thyroid lesions. This obviated a vibration source external to the neck, and they were able to distinguish 10 papillary carcinomas from 43 other thyroid lesions based on the stiffness.

Acoustic radiation force impulse (AFRI) imaging uses short-duration ultrasound pulses (0.03 to 0.4 ms) to create tissue movement/displacement and recovery, which is recorded with ultrasound correlation or Doppler ultrasound. There are no clinical studies of the head and neck, but AFRI has been used to better identify isoechoic lesions within the liver, stiffness of the heart myocardium, solid versus cystic lesions in the pancreas, and luminal intestinal lesions. Certainly, there is a potential value within the head and neck. One of the early concerns of ARFI is heat produced at the transducer and tissue being examined. Advances in AFRI beam sequencing and parallel imaging

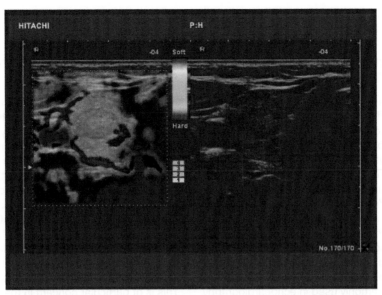

Fig. 2. Elastography images of thyroid nodule. (*Courtesy of* Signotics Inc, USA [Web site: superdupertech.com/2009/05]; with permission.)

have shortened acquisition time and reduced transducer heating significantly, reducing this concern.[7]

COMBINING LIGHT AND SOUND IN PHOTOACOUSTIC IMAGING

Photoacoustic imaging (PAI) was designed to detect tissue vascularity more precisely. In PAI, a nonionizing laser targets human chromophores, such as hemoglobin and melanin, heating the tissue and causing expansion then contraction, which, in turn, gives off detectable ultrasonic waves. These ultrasonic waves are collected by an ultrasound transducer and produce an ultra-sound image. In a limited study of 3 patients with port-wine stains, Kolkman[8] in 2008 demonstrated advantages in more precisely determining vascular layer and lesion depths of these vascular lesions. Nanoparticles, such as gold nanorods, shells, and cages, are particularly sensitive to light stimulation. They are being used to increase

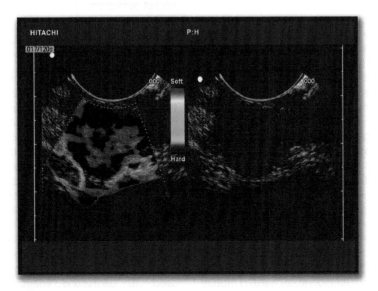

Fig. 3. Malignant upper mediastinal lymph node in esophageal carcinoma. (*Courtesy of* Hitachi Medical Systems, Europe [Web site: http://www.hitachi-medical-systems.eu/products-and-services/ct.html]; with permission.)

sensitivity of PAI,[9] but there are no clinical studies specific to the head and neck as yet.

CONTRAST-ENHANCING ULTRASOUND WITH MICROBUBBLES

Doppler imaging does not show capillary blood flow. Using 3- to 5-micron air bubbles or microbubbles injected intravenously to reflect the ultrasound waves provides increased vascular detail not available with Doppler imaging. Differences in microcirculation have been shown to be useful in differentiating metastatic from benign cervical lymph nodes (Zenk, 2007).[10] Examples of current commercially available microbubble contrast agents used within the head and neck include Sonovue and Sonazoid. Sonovue consists of 2.5-micron sulfur hexafluoride microbubbles stabilized with phospholipids and lasting in suspension up to 6 hours. It is commonly used in echocardiography but has also been used in imaging micrometastases in cervical lymph nodes. Sonazoid consists of perfluorocarbon with a surfactant stabilizing shell, which, when injected intravascularly, is taken up by the macrophages of the reticuloendothelial system. In the animal model, it has been injected at the tumor site to detect sentinel lymph node metastasis with 90% sensitivity as compared with 81% sensitivity in lymphoscintigraphy.[11] Both canine and porcine animal studies have found contrast-enhanced ultrasound effective in sentinel lymph node biopsy within the head and neck.[12,13] Without contrast, high-resolution ultrasound detected only 45.8% of positive neck sentinel lymph nodes in a recent large clinical melanoma study.[14]

Beyond enhancing ultrasonic images, microbubbles can have target ligands on their surface so that they are concentrated in a specific anatomic area of interest and may contain drugs for targeted delivery or even DNA plasmids to be released for gene therapy. Microbubbles can be used for thrombolysis by enhancing enzymatic thrombolytic action. Clinical trials are currently under way using mechanical pressure waves generated by transcranial ultrasound to break up clots (sonothrombolysis) and increase penetration of the thrombolytic enzyme recombinant tissue plasminogen activator (tPA).[15] Tsivgoulis and colleagues[16] performed a meta-analysis on the safety and efficacy of sonothrombolysis and found that it was not associated with any increased risk of "rebleed" and that there was a higher recanalization rate with the addition of microbubbles than with tPA alone. Ultrasound-stimulated motion of microbubbles enhances permeability across cell membranes, and endothelium provides better

drug delivery which is likely to prove useful in the future for other drugs.[17]

HIGH-INTENSITY FOCUSED ULTRASOUND SURGERY

High-intensity focused ultrasound (HIFU) surgery is being developed for clinical use in hepatic, renal, prostate, and intracranial surgery, but the head and neck is certainly a possible future application as strategies to limit collateral damage in adjacent tissue are refined. HIFU creates tissue destruction through heating up the tissue and creating a coagulation necrosis with a focal acoustic lens at very low frequencies (1 to 1.5 MHz). Because of the focused nature of the ultrasound beam, the heat gradient for surrounding tissues drops off rapidly, but there can be difficulty with often cigar-shaped focal zones and damage to nearby tissue. This is of particular concern in the head and neck, because of the close proximity of critical structures. Further increasing the intensity of the HIFU can cause cavitations within the cells resulting in cell destruction. Histotripsy is an ultrasound-based strategy in the renal model that uses high-frequency ultrasound to produce cavitations with minimal heat production, thereby minimizing the risk of thermal damage to adjacent tissue.[18] In an attempt to better monitor the thermal damage to surrounding brain tissue, Jolesz and colleagues[19] have successfully used 1.5-tesla MRI that can detect changes of 3° in conjunction with HIFU applied intracranially. HIFU has also been used to occlude renal arteries in an animal model[20] and has potential usefulness in hemostasis and vessel occlusion.

THREE-DIMENSIONAL ULTRASOUND IMAGING WITHIN THE HEAD AND NECK

With an intrauterine assessment of facial abnormalities, Tonni and colleagues[21] in 2005 found three-dimensional (3D) ultrasound imaging superior to 2D in the intrauterine fetal detection of cleft lip and palate defects and advocate its routine use for screening in the second trimester of pregnancy. Imaging of the head and neck commonly uses 3D reconstructions in computed tomography (CT) and MRI for vascular tumors, reconstruction after facial trauma, and complex masses. Both 3- and 4D (using time or video as the fourth dimension) ultrasound images are potentially useful for head and neck tumor assessment and detection. In a very limited study, Carraro and colleagues[22] used 3D ultrasound images enhanced with contrast microbubbles to characterize the vasculature and volume of 4 benign and 4 malignant thyroid nodules, demonstrating a higher internal vasculature in the malignant (52.3% ± 15.7%) than the benign (14.3% ± 5.3%). Zhou and colleagues[23] calculated a tumor vascularity index using a combination of 2D and 3D Doppler ultrasound of 87 patients with laryngeal carcinoma to predict cervical lymph node metastases and found a 98% specificity and 95% sensitivity.

TECHNIQUES TO SUPPRESS IMAGE ARTIFACT

Spatial compounding (SonoCT; Philips Healthcare, Andover, MA, USA) scans a lesion at different angles in real time to minimize artifact. It can "compound" up to 9 images to eliminate scatter artifact and give a more accurate image. Harmonic imaging (THI) uses integer multiples of the tissues' fundamental frequency based on the principle that these harmonic integers or overtones increase initially with increasing depth of tissue. Their increase in strength with depth lessens the effect of image artifact. Manipulations of the harmonics using second harmonics and broadband inversion techniques (Ensemble THI) further reduce image artifact. Using the fundamental frequency of microbubbles along with THI has an synergistic effect on image quality and has been called contrast harmonic imaging. Techniques to improve image quality are likely to be developed in the future.[24]

REAL-TIME IMAGE-GUIDED SURGERY

Helbig and colleagues[25] have developed a prototype for use in real-time image-guided navigational surgery, which may prove useful in soft-tissue surgery of the neck. This would provide the ability to surgically navigate from the current anatomic relationships, not relying on the preoperative relationships as in currently used CT and MRI navigational systems. There is also the potential to combine CT and ultrasound in image-guided navigational surgery for added information, because CT and MRI are currently combined in specific surgical cases.

INCREASING USE OF ULTRASOUND

With the increasing popularity of ultrasonography performed by the clinician directly caring for the patient, there will be a demand for smaller machines with better imaging. Future modifications to improve image quality similar to Harmonic imaging and "compounding images" to reduce artifact will only accelerate ultrasound's clinical use. Use of 3D and 4D ultrasound will likely expand, but currently is limited to complex images. Supplementing the physical exam in

real-time to include more information on benign versus malignant lesions, is where current emerging technology in ultrasound is likely to make a significant impact. Using objective palpation of tumor or lymph node stiffness coupled with additional tissue vascular detail using microbubbles would undoubtedly enhance the ability to distinguish benign from malignant. Success in the animal model point to the potential use of microbubbles and ultrasound in sentinel lymph node biopsy. Combining imaging modalities such as MRI with Ultrasound and Laser stimulation to provide better ultrasound imaging (Photoacoustic imaging) is providing better information than these entities used alone.

Dramatic advancement is likely in the realm of therapeutic intervention. Although the promise of coagulating bleeders with HIFU has great appeal, this area has been researched for some time and has yet to be perfected. The most impressive possibilities are in the area of targeted microbubble delivery of drugs and DNA plasmids. The ability to attach ligands to microbubbles and have relatively precise delivery of therapeutic medical interventions coupled with ultrasound's ability to increase cell penetration holds great promise for the therapeutic use of ultrasound.

REFERENCES

1. James JA, Dalton GA, Bullen MA, et al. The ultrasonic treatment of Meniere's disease. J Laryngol Otol 1960;74:730–57.
2. Hong Y, Liu X, Li Z, et al. Real-time ultrasound elastography in the differential diagnosis of benign and malignant thyroid nodules. J Ultrasound Med 2009; 28(7):861–7.
3. Rago T, Santini F, Scutari M, et al. Elastography: new developments in ultrasound for predicting malignancy in thyroid nodules. J Clin Endocrinol Metab 2007;92(8):2917–22.
4. Asteria C, Giovanardi A, Pizzocaro A, et al. US-elastography in the differential diagnosis of benign and malignant thyroid nodules. Thyroid 2008;18(5): 523–31.
5. Lyshchik A, Higashi T, Asato R, et al. Cervical lymph node metastases: diagnosis at sonoelastography–initial experience. Radiology 2007;243(1):258–67.
6. Dighe M, Bae U, Richardson ML, et al. Differential diagnosis of thyroid nodules with US elastography using carotid artery pulsation. Radiology 2008; 248(2):662–9.
7. Hsu SJ, Bouchard RR, Dumont DM, et al. Novel acoustic radiation force impulse imaging methods for visualization of rapidly moving tissue. Ultrason Imaging 2009;31(3):183–200.

8. Kolkman RG, Mulder MJ, Glade CP, et al. Photoacoustic imaging of port-wine stains. Lasers Surg Med 2008;40(3):178–82.

9. Yang X, Stein EW, Ashkenazi S, et al. Nanoparticles for photoacoustic imaging. Wiley Interdiscip Rev Nanomed Nanobiotechnol 2009;1(4):360–8.

10. Zenk J, Bozzato A, Hornung J, et al. Neck lymph nodes: prediction by computer-assisted contrast medium analysis? Ultrasound Med Biol 2007;33: 246–53.

11. Stramare R, Scagliori E, Mannucci M, et al. The role of contrast-enhanced gray-scale ultrasonography in the differential diagnosis of superficial lymph nodes. Ultrasound Q 2010;26(1):45–51.

12. Lurie DM, Seguin B, Schneider PD, et al. Contrast-assisted ultrasound for sentinel lymph node detection in spontaneously arising canine head and neck tumors. Invest Radiol 2006;41(4):415–21.

13. Curry JM, Bloedon E, Malloy KM, et al. Ultrasound-guided contrast-enhanced sentinel node biopsy of the head and neck in a porcine model. Otolaryngol Head Neck Surg 2007;137(5):735–41.

14. Sanki A, Uren RF, Moncrieff M, et al. Targeted high-resolution ultrasound is not an effective substitute for sentinel lymph node biopsy in patients with primary cutaneous melanoma. J Clin Oncol 2009;27(33): 5614–9.

15. Rubiera M, Alexandrov AV. Sonothrombolysis in the management of acute ischemic stroke. Am J Cardiovasc Drugs 2010;10(1):5–10.

16. Tsivgoulis G, Eggers J, Ribo M, et al. Safety and efficacy of ultrasound-enhanced thrombolysis: a comprehensive review and meta-analysis of randomized and nonrandomized studies. Stroke 2010;41(2): 280–7.

17. Stride EP, Coussios CC. Cavitation and contrast: the use of bubbles in ultrasound imaging and therapy. Proc Inst Mech Eng H 2010;224(2):171–91.

18. Klatte T, Marberger M. High-intensity focused ultrasound for the treatment of renal masses: current status and future potential. Curr Opin Urol 2009; 19(2):188–91.

19. Jagannathan J, Sanghvi N, Crum L, et al. High-intensity focused ultrasound surgery of the brain: part 1–A historical perspective with modern applications. Neurosurgery 2009;64(2):201–10 [discussion: 210–1].

20. Rove KO, Sullivan KF, Crawford ED. High-intensity focused ultrasound: ready for primetime. Urol Clin North Am 2010;37(1):27–35 [table of contents].

21. Tonni G, Centini G, Rosignoli L. Prenatal screening for fetal face and clefting in a prospective study on low-risk population: can 3- and 4-dimensional ultrasound enhance visualization and detection rate? Oral Surg Oral Med Oral Pathol Oral Radiol Endod 2005;100(4):420–6.

22. Carraro R, Molinari F, Deandrea M, et al. Characterization of thyroid nodules by 3-D contrast-enhanced ultrasound imaging. Conf Proc IEEE Eng Med Biol Soc 2008;2008:2229–32.

23. Zhou J, Shang-Yong Z, Ruo-Chuan L, et al. Vascularity index of laryngeal cancer derived from 3-D ultrasound: a predicting factor for the in vivo assessment of cervical lymph node status. Ultrasound Med Biol 2009;35(10):1596–600.

24. Hoefer M. Ultrasound teaching manual. 2nd edition. Theme; 2005. p.120.

25. Helbig M, Krysztoforski K, Krowick P, et al. Development of prototype for navigated real-time sonography for the head and neck region. Head Neck 2008;30(2):215–21.

Head and Neck Ultrasound: Applications Relevant to Anesthesia and Intensive Care Medicine

James S. Green, MBBS, FRCA, Ban C.H. Tsui, MD, FRCPC*

KEYWORDS

- Ultrasound • Airway • Regional • Anesthesia • ENT
- Vascular access

The use of ultrasound imaging in clinical practice is becoming more widely adopted. It is currently used in many centers to facilitate vascular access and regional anesthesia in addition to the traditional role of diagnostic imaging. Using real-time ultrasonography, one can guide the needle directly toward the target (nerve for regional anesthesia, or vessel for vascular access) under visualization. Ultrasonography may help the clinician to avoid critical structures in the path of the needle, therefore potentially improving success while reducing complications. The use of ultrasonography in regional anesthesia has the additional benefit of allowing visualization of accurate distribution of local anesthetic.[1] Recent reports involving sonography of both the neck[2] and the upper airway[3] demonstrate its clinical potential at these anatomic locations.

As time progresses it is important to regularly review areas of ultrasound practice. In this review, we explore the use of ultrasound imaging of the head and neck relevant to anesthesia and intensive care medicine.

We attempt to answer pertinent questions such as: Does the use of ultrasonography have the potential to increase the sensitivity and specificity for prediction of difficult airway? Could it offer assistance for airway procedures such as percutaneous tracheostomy and awake fiberoptic intubation? Can the success and safety of regional anesthesia of the head and neck be improved with ultrasonography? And will the use of ultrasonography offer tangible clinical benefit in these areas that can be exploited in day-to-day clinical practice by the majority of anesthesiologists? The use of ultrasound for central venous catheter (CVC) placement is topical and we provide an overview of imaging for internal jugular and subclavian vein cannulation.

ULTRASONOGRAPHY IN AIRWAY ASSESSMENT AND MANAGEMENT
Percutaneous Tracheostomy

Percutaneous tracheostomy is frequently performed in the intensive care unit (ICU) setting. Many complications have been reported, including hemorrhage from local vessels and tracheal stenosis due to cranial placement of the tracheostomy.[4] The use of ultrasonography allows avoidance of vascular structures,[4,5] identification of

A version of this article was previously published in the September 2010 issue of *Anesthesiology Clinics of North America*.

Funding support: B.C.H.T. is supported by a Clinical Scholar Award from Alberta Heritage Foundation for Medical Research, Edmonton, Alberta, Canada, and a Career Scientist Award from the Canadian Anesthesiologists' Society/Abbott Laboratories, Toronto, Ontario, Canada.

Disclosure: The authors have nothing to disclose.

Department of Anesthesiology and Pain Medicine, University of Alberta, 8-120 Clinical Sciences Building, Edmonton, Alberta T6G 2G3, Canada

* Corresponding author.

E-mail address: btsui@ualberta.ca

ultrasound.theclinics.com

the midline,[4,5] and identification of tracheal rings to avoid high (cranial) placement, and lowers the risk of laryngotracheal stenosis.[4,6]

In one observational study, ultrasound images of the anterior neck were obtained from 50 volunteers.[4] The distance between the caudal border of the cricoid cartilage and the second tracheal ring was found to be variable across subjects (range 9.7–29.7 mm). Consequently, it was proposed that the use of ultrasonography could be useful in accurately identifying the second to third cervical level for tracheostomy. The sonoanatomy of a longitudinal view of the larynx and trachea has been previously described (**Fig. 1**).[7]

An autopsy study compared the use of "blind" versus ultrasound-guided percutaneous dilatational tracheostomy (PDT) in ICU patients.[6] In 5 of 15 (33%) patients from the blind group the tracheostomy tube was found to be placed between the cricoid cartilage and the first tracheal ring (cranial misplacement). Cranial misplacement was not seen in the 11 patients for whom ultrasound imaging was used, indicating that the use of ultrasonography may reduce or eliminate misplacement.

Sustic and Zupan[7] used ultrasound imaging in 30 patients prior to percutaneous tracheostomy to assist in identification of vessels proximal to the puncture site in addition to location of the midline and level of tracheal puncture. The tracheal midline, thyroid isthmus, and level for needle insertion were identifiable in all patients. Anterior jugular veins were identified and electively ligated in 15 patients. "Vulnerable" carotid or brachiocephalic arteries were identified in 4 patients.

Case reports on the use of ultrasonography for percutaneous tracheostomy following anterior cervical spine fixation[8] and in an obese patient[9] have indicated its potential usefulness in these challenging cases. The use of ultrasound imaging before insertion of percutaneous tracheostomy has the potential to improve clinical care by reducing the associated complications, but further studies are required for confirmation.

The use of ultrasound in the emergency cricothyroidotomy situation has not been described, but if access to ultrasound was at hand then real-time use by a skilled operator could potentially increase success. Ultrasound can also be used to identify the cricothyroid membrane in the neck of a patient with a potentially difficult airway prior to attempted awake fibre-optic endotracheal intubation. This can be performed while waiting for onset of topical anesthesia to the airway and is therefore a practical option for more widespread use. Marking the cricothyroid membrane can provide an readily identifiable landmark to aid insertion of needle cricothyroidotomy if airway control is later lost and emergency cricothyroidotomy required.

The 4th national audit project from the Royal College of Anaesthetists in the UK highlighted a 60% failure rate associated with emergency cricothyroidotomy.[10] This certainly leaves room for improvement, and the role of ultrasound in this area therefore warrants further evaluation in conjunction with other developments such a recently described electrical stimulation technique for identifying the tracheal lumen.[11]

Visualization of the Epiglottis and Larynx

A sublingual approach for direct ultrasound visualization of the epiglottis was proposed by Tsui and Hui; however, further investigation revealed that the structure initially thought to be the epiglottis was in fact the hyoid bone.[12] Of the anatomic structures of interest, the epiglottis is suspended

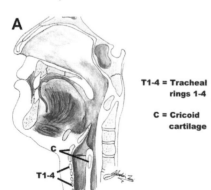
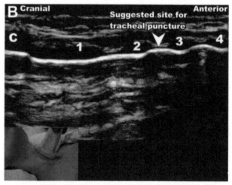

T1-4 = Tracheal rings 1-4

C = Cricoid cartilage

Fig. 1. (A) Regional anatomy and (B) ultrasound image (HFL38 6–13 MHz 38 mm footprint, Sonosite M-turbo; Bothell, WA, USA) of cricoid cartilage and tracheal rings using midline longitudinal scanning plane at the level of the larynx on the anterior neck (probe placement in *inset*). The cricoid cartilage and the first 4 tracheal rings are seen, and the ultrasound shadow cast posteriorly from each of these rings aids with their identification. Overlying vessels, if identified due to their compressibility, will appear as hypoechoic structures, round to oval if seen in cross section or straight if seen longitudinally.

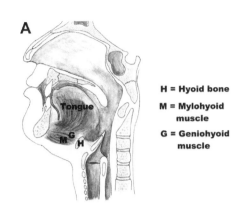

H = Hyoid bone

M = Mylohyoid muscle

G = Geniohyoid muscle

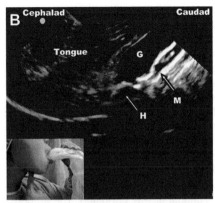

Fig. 2. Sublingual ultrasound imaging (C11 7–4 MHz curved, Sonosite M-turbo; Bothell, WA, USA) fails to capture the epiglottis due to the presence of air, a poor ultrasound medium. As labeled in the regional anatomy drawing (A) and the image (B), the hyoid bone and its functional musculature is clearly identified *arrows*.

in air and the esophagus is posterior to the air-filled trachea (**Fig. 2**). Air is a poor ultrasound medium, appearing as a hyperechoic artifact that does not afford visualization of deeper structures.

Transverse and longitudinal transcutaneous imaging approaches have also been described for visualizing the epiglottis.[13,14] The appearance of the epiglottis can be captured through the hyothyroid window (between the hyoid bone and the thyroid cartilage) and its average anteroposterior thickness was found to be 2.49 ± 0.13 mm.[14] In transverse axis, the epiglottis appears as a curvilinear hypoechoic structure beneath an echogenic pre-epiglottic space and with dorsal acoustic shadowing.[14] For the longitudinal axis, Prasad and colleagues[13] use a parasagittal approach 2 cm lateral to the midline to identify the epiglottis cephalad and caudad to the hypoechoic mass of

the hyoid bone. A hyperechogenicity adjacent to the epiglottis is described as the "mucocutaneous surface of the epiglottis due to the formation of the air-mucosa interface." This group has recently published an observational study to evaluate the feasibility of airway sonography (by an experienced sonographer) and to determine the optimal scanning technique.[3] Due to acoustic shadowing from the hyoid bone, a parasagittal view of the epiglottis was only obtained by 71% of studied subjects. Singh and colleagues[3] used tongue protrusion and swallowing to confirm the identity of the epiglottis as a discrete mobile structure inferior to the base of the tongue. Reproducing such a clear view of the epiglottis in the parasagittal view can be challenging, as demonstrated by the authors' efforts at this technique (**Fig. 3**).[13] Also describing a parasagittal approach, Garel and

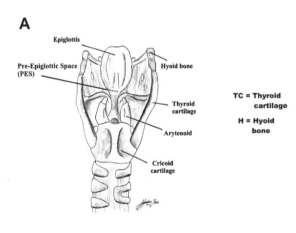

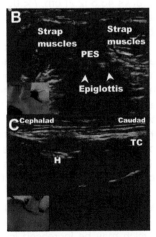

Fig. 3. (A) Relevant regional anatomy for visualizing the epiglottis (posterior view) and images captured (HFL38 6–13 MHz 38 mm footprint, Sonosite M-turbo; Bothell, WA, USA) using (B) transverse and (C) parasagittal longitudinal scanning planes at the anterior aspect of the neck. The photos in the insets show the corresponding probe placement. Although a similar approach to that of Prasad and colleagues[13] was used here for illustrating the parasagittal view, the investigators had difficulty identifying the epiglottis in this view.

colleagues[15] describe the epiglottis as appearing hyperechoic during laryngeal ultrasonography. Only the subhyoid portion was visible due to surrounding air obscuring the margin.

Epiglottal and pre-epiglottal edema (enlargement) due to pharyngolaryngeal infection has recently been diagnosed with ultrasonography.[16] A moderate increase in thickness of the epiglottis (3.2 mm as compared with 2.49 ± 0.13 mm found by Werner and colleagues[14]) was similar to the fiberoptic finding of moderate swelling. Ultrasonography to aid the diagnosis of epiglottitis may prove to be a useful tool for identification and management of this critical airway condition. The authors could not locate any trials evaluating the use of ultrasonography in epiglottitis for this review. The benefits of the use of ultrasonography in these situations—rapidity, noninvasiveness, and comfort—may speed its evaluation and clinical implementation.

Laryngeal ultrasonography has been used to investigate lymphangioma, laryngeal atresia, and papillomatosis, as well as subglottic stenosis and hemangioma.[15,17]

Prediction of Airway Difficulties

Ezri and colleagues[18] report on the use of ultrasonography to predict difficult intubation in obese patients. An abundance of pretracheal soft tissue (from the skin to the anterior aspect of the trachea) at the level of the vocal cords was found to be a predictor of difficult laryngoscopy. Patients in whom laryngoscopy was difficult had more pretracheal soft tissue (mean [SD] 28 [2.7] mm vs 17.5 [1.8] mm; $P<.001$) and a greater neck circumference (50 [3.8] vs 43.5 [2.2] cm; $P<.001$). Of note, 7 of 9 patients in whom laryngoscopy was difficult had a history of obstructive sleep apnea, which may have been associated with the greater neck circumference and increased pretracheal soft tissue. Four years later a group consisting of some of the same investigators published a study with similar methodology in the Unites States and reported conflicting results.[19]

Although Tsui and Hui[12] found sublingual ultrasonography to be of little value for assessing the epiglottis (see **Fig. 2**), they have observed that this imaging may have merit for predicting airway difficulties using the identification of the hyoid bone as a landmark.[20] In 1993, Chou and Wu[21] described a new predictive factor, hyomandibular distance, which may be increased in those with a difficult airway. Defined as the vertical distance between the upper margin of the hyoid bone and lower margin of the mandible, hyomandibular distance can be long for 2 reasons: a caudally

displaced hyoid bone or a short mandibular ramus. Successful intubation by direct laryngoscopy requires alignment of the oral and pharyngeal axes followed by anterior displacement of the tongue and epiglottis. Caudal displacement of the hyoid bone may cause a larger proportion of the tongue to be situated in the hypopharynx.[22] Caudal displacement of the larynx would likely hinder the ability to visualize the hyoid bone. Its subsequent identification with sublingual ultrasonography may help predict difficult laryngoscopy and/or intubation. In a pilot study of 100 elective surgical patients, Hui and Tsui[20] (preliminary data reported) found that failure to identify the hyoid bone with sublingual ultrasonography predicted a laryngoscopic view of III or greater (11 patients having Grade III–IV view) with 72.7% sensitivity, 96.6% specificity, and 72.7% positive predictive value. These data show an improvement over other tests for predicting laryngoscopic view of greater than III: Mallampati score had 36.4% sensitivity, 87.6% specificity, and 26.7% positive predictive value, thyromental distance less than 6 cm had 9.1% sensitivity and 100% specificity, and decreased neck extension had 36.4% sensitivity and 88.8% specificity.

Confirmation of Correct Airway Device Placement

Ultrasonography has been used to confirm endotracheal tube placement in adults, both indirectly by visualization of diaphragmatic and pleural movement[23] and directly by visualization of a stylet or fluid-filled cuff.[24–26] In pediatrics, endotracheal tube placement has also been confirmed sonographically through visualization of the trachea and cords, with widening of the cords viewed on passage of the endotracheal tube.[27] Esophageal intubation was also seen in the paratracheal space in the same study. In cadavers, real-time transcricothyroid ultrasonography had high sensitivity (97%) and specificity (100%) for detecting esophageal endotracheal tube placement.[28] In another study, all of 5 patients with esophageal tube placement were identified as having such using transtracheal ultrasonography.[29] The correct placement of a double-lumen tube[30] and laryngeal mask airway (if filled with water)[26] have also been described.

Using longitudinal scanning, the appearance of endotracheal intubation has been described as a "snow storm" between 2 hyperechoic lines depicting the anterior and posterior laryngeal walls. This "snow storm" does not appear on esophageal intubation, and there may also be the appearance of movement posterior to the 2 laryngeal lines.[28] Static imaging after intubation has shown to be far inferior to dynamic (real-time) imaging for detecting esophageal intubation.[28] Transverse scanning with the probe placed at a 45° angle over the cricothyroid membrane results in an image of a curved thyroid cartilage superficially with the carotid arteries and internal jugular veins on either side.[29] Esophageal intubation produces a striking image with a clearly visible curved hyperechoic line with distal shadowing.

Current methods to confirm airway device placement include direct visualization of passage of the endotracheal tube between the vocal cords, end-tidal carbon dioxide monitoring, clinical examination, and bronchoscopy in the case of double-lumen tube placement. When combined, these methods are effective at detecting esophageal intubation and are readily accessible in the operating room. One disadvantage of relying on these methods is that gastric insufflation can occur before recognition of esophageal intubation. Ultrasonography could have a role in confirming endotracheal intubation, with the advantage of preventing gastric insufflation in the event of esophageal intubation; this may be particularly useful when passage of the endotracheal tube is not directly visualized (such as in Cormack Lehane Grade 3 or 4 view). Further research is required to fully evaluate the clinical impact of the routine use of ultrasonography for this indication.

Other Applications of Ultrasonography Related to the Airway

The presence of airway edema after oropharyngeal surgery may result in postextubation stridor. In an effort to overcome the limitations of the cuff-leak test, the ability of ultrasonography to predict postextubation stridor has been evaluated by using ultrasound-measured air-column widths.[31] In a study of 51 consecutive planned extubations, the air-leak volume (300 vs 25 mL) and air-column widths (6.4 vs 4.5 mm) were significantly less in patients with stridor (rate of 7.8%). These investigators placed the ultrasound probe transversely on the cricothyroid membrane while the patient's balloon cuff was both inflated and deflated. The air-column width was defined as the width of air that passed through the vocal cords, and this width noticeably enlarged on cuff deflation in patients who did not develop stridor.

Endobronchial ultrasonography has shown to be successful for distinguishing between compression of the airway and infiltration by tumor in patients with central thoracic malignancies,[32,33] for assessing expiratory airway collapse in chronic obstructive pulmonary disease and tracheomalacia,[34] and for assessing bronchial wall thickening in patients

with asthma.[35] Endobronchial ultrasonography is not readily available for use by anesthesiologists in the majority of centers, limiting the scope for use. However, this is an area for future research to determine whether the use of endobronchial ultrasonography by anesthesiologists can direct management decisions and influence outcomes in situations with a critical airway problem.

Other uses of ultrasonography have been described, including the detection of a nonrecurrent laryngeal nerve in ENT patients,[36–38] and the detection of postoperative laryngeal nerve palsy using B-mode and color Doppler.[38,39]

APPLICATION OF ULTRASONOGRAPHY FOR NERVE BLOCKS IN ENT
Deep Cervical Plexus Block

Deep cervical plexus blocks have been used for anterior neck procedures such as awake carotid endarterectomy, lymph node biopsy, and plastic surgery.[40] Several ultrasound-guided approaches to the cervical plexus have been described.[2] An injection into the longus capitis at the level of C4 has shown to achieve blockade of the C2 to C5 nerve roots (located in a groove between the longus capitis and scalenus medius muscles) and of the sympathetic trunk (located on the anteromedial surface of the longus capitis muscle).[41] After performing an anatomic study in 28 cadavers, Usui and colleagues[41] determined that the injection position was localized to the site where a cranially directed ultrasound scan, initially focused on the scalenus anterior and longus capitis muscle at the level of C6, captured the point where the scalenus anterior muscle tapered off at either C3 or C4. Computed tomography showed that although confined to the muscle, the local anesthetic infiltrated into the neighboring nerve structures. An important finding from this article is that that the deep cervical plexus was not located in the interscalene groove, and that selective deep cervical plexus block can be performed in the groove between the longus capitis and scalenus medius (Fig. 4).

The cervical nerve roots travel in the sulcus between the anterior and posterior tubercles of the transverse processes, and course inferoposterior to the vertebral artery. The roots appear posterior to the anterior tubercles using a transverse view, but posterior to the vertebral artery using a longitudinal plane.[2] Identification of the vertebral artery and transverse processes of C2 to C4 allows cervical plexus block posterior to the artery.[2,40] Scanning caudally from the mastoid process, the level of the C2 transverse process and nerve root are identified through recognition of the loop that

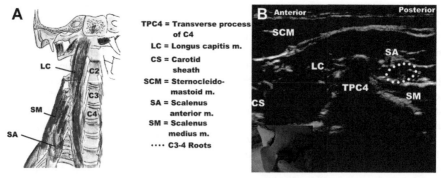

Fig. 4. (*A*) Regional anatomy and (*B*) ultrasound image (HFL38 6–13 MHz 38 mm footprint, Sonosite M-turbo; Bothell, WA, USA) with the probe placed at the anterolateral position at the approximate level of C4. The photo in the inset shows corresponding probe placement. The longus capitis muscle is captured anterolateral to the carotid sheath.

the vertebral artery makes as it travels between the foramen of C2 and C1. Subsequently, 3 injections may be performed between C1 and C4. Compared with blind landmark-based approaches, ultrasonography allows appraisal of both plexus depth (through location of the vertebral artery) and craniocaudal level (via the starting point of the arterial loop). **Fig. 5**[40] shows an image of the vertebral artery at the level of C2 to C3, and although the "loop" is not captured, the pulsatile artery is identified with ultrasound. It must be noted that these approaches are advanced ultrasound-guided techniques. Further evaluation of their safety is warranted prior to recommendation for widespread clinical use.

The use of ultrasound-guided high interscalene blocks and deep cervical plexus blocks to provide local anesthesia for carotid endarterectomy have also been described.[42,43] Using high-resolution ultrasonography, Roessel and colleagues[43] identified the upper portion (C4) of the brachial plexus, 1.5 ± 0.2 cm lateral to the common carotid artery, and although they used 20 mL of local anesthetic for the blocks as little as 5 mL was shown to

surround the plexus. This indicates that ultrasonography may enable accurate placement of smaller doses of local anesthetic, thereby limiting the risk of systemic toxicity.

Kefalianakis and colleagues[42] reported high success with surgical anesthesia using ultrasound-guided block of the deep cervical plexus, combined with additional subcutaneous injection for superficial cervical plexus block and sedation. The local anesthetic for these deep blocks was injected between the scalenus anterior and sternocleidomastoid muscle at the level of the carotid bifurcation.

Nerve Blocks for Awake Fiberoptic Intubation

At present, there is no ultrasound-guided nerve block specifically described for awake fiberoptic intubation. However, ultrasonography may be useful when performing several techniques for providing airway anesthesia. These methods include sensory nerve blockade or application of local anesthetics to the respiratory mucosa via cricothyroid needle puncture.

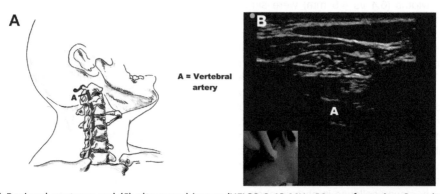

Fig. 5. (*A*) Regional anatomy and (*B*) ultrasound image (HFL38 6–13 MHz 38 mm footprint, Sonosite M-turbo; Bothell, WA, USA) of the vertebral artery at the level of C2 to C3. The pulsatile artery was easily identified with ultrasonography.

To provide anesthesia for the supraglottic larynx, the superior laryngeal nerve block can be used, while the cricothyroid injection has been shown to be effective for subglottic structures.[44] In clinical practice, the glossopharyngeal nerve block has also been shown to be effective for obtunding the gag reflex, although this approach is used less frequently. Because approaching the glossopharyngeal nerve via the styloid approach places the needle in close proximity to many blood vessels, it is anticipated that this risk may be reduced if direct visualization using ultrasound is used.

In a cadaveric study, the proximity of the superior laryngeal nerve to the greater cornu of the hyoid bone was demonstrated.[45] The mean distance from internal superior laryngeal nerve to the greater horn of the hyoid bone in a craniocaudal direction was found to be 2.4 mm. **Fig. 6** illustrates an image of the hyoid bone and the relevant anatomy for the superior laryngeal block, demonstrating that ultrasonography could facilitate deposition of local anesthetic at the superolateral aspect of the hyoid bone.

Ideally, the dual aims of airway anesthesia are to abolish sensory innervation and the afferent limbs of protective airway reflexes to facilitate endotracheal intubation. Nevertheless, the effectiveness of sensory nerve blocks has been compared with topical local anesthetic in spray and nebulized form.[46,47] Although patient comfort and hemodynamic stability may vary between the different approaches, intubating conditions are not any different.[46]

Alveolar Nerve Block

Ultrasonography for inferior alveolar nerve blockade for pulpal anesthesia (at the mandibular teeth) has been compared with the conventional technique in a randomized controlled study.[48]

For this intraoral block, the transducer head with needle guide was placed on the medial aspect of the mandibular ramus to identify the mandibular ramus, the medial pterygoid and masseter muscles, and the inferior alveolar artery (using color Doppler). After localizing the artery, the needle was positioned in the guide and directed into the pterygomandibular space toward the neurovascular bundle. There was no difference in outcome between the ultrasound-guided and the blind technique, despite accurate placement of local anesthetic under imaging.

Superficial Trigeminal Nerve Blocks

Peripheral blocks of the terminal branches of the trigeminal nerve can be used for surgical repair of soft tissue injury of the face. Failure rates to achieve full anesthesia using traditional blocks of the trigeminal nerve have been reported in the region of 22%.[49] Infraorbital nerve blockade can be used to provide analgesia following surgery for cleft lip repair.[50] However, adult landmarks used to perform infraorbital nerve blocks are absent or difficult to palpate in the neonate. Facial foramina can be localized accurately and reliably using ultrasonography,[48,51] and this may provide an opportunity to improve success in these blocks. Recently, Tsui[51] described an ultrasound approach to locate the supraorbital, infraorbital, and mental foramina. Using a high-resolution, short-footprint linear transducer, a disruption of the continuity of bone in the vicinity of each foramen is used to identify the respective foramen (**Fig. 7**).

Greater Occipital Nerve Block

Local anesthetic block of the greater occipital nerve can be useful for certain neurosurgical procedures, for example, pin insertion for craniotomy, as well as

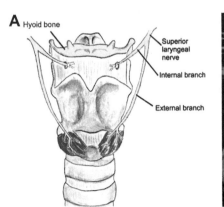
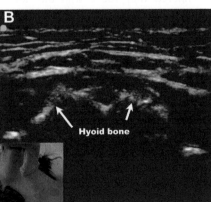

Fig. 6. (*A*) Regional anatomy and (*B*) ultrasound image (HFL38 6–13 MHz 38 mm footprint, Sonosite M-turbo; Bothell, WA, USA) capturing hyoid bone, which may also be suitable for guidance of superior laryngeal nerve blockade (*arrows*).

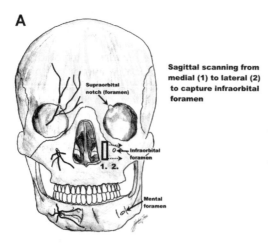
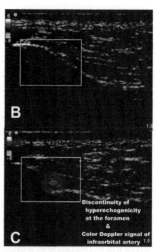

Fig. 7. (*A*) Skull with foramen and the respective nerves, and a representation of the scanning plane and direction (1. to 2.) used to localize the foramen as a discontinuity of the hyperechogenicity of the bone. Ultrasound images (HFL38 6–13 MHz 38 mm footprint, Sonosite M-turbo; Bothell, WA, USA) are medial to the foramen (*B*) and at the foraminal position (*C*), where the discontinuity is clearly depicted and the artery is captured with color Doppler.

for the treatment of chronic pain mediated by the greater occipital nerve. A recent cadaveric study compared 2 techniques of ultrasound guidance, using both the traditional block site and a selective approach at a proximal location where the nerve curls around the lower border of the obliquus capitis inferior muscle after emerging below the posterior arch of the atlas.[52] A transverse midline orientation is initially used to identify the external occipital protuberance. A caudal scan is used to identify the spinous process of C2 by its bifid appearance. A lateral rotation of the transducer is used to locate the obliquus capitis inferior muscle. The nerve is identified during its cranial course where it lies superficial to the muscle. Reported success of the simulated block, defined by spread of dye to the nerve, was 80% using the traditional landmarks compared with 100% with the new selective technique.

ULTRASOUND FOR CVC PLACEMENT

The American Society of Echocardiography and Society of Cardiovascular Anesthesiologists has recommended guidelines for performing ultrasound guided vascular cannulation.[53] They recommend the use of real-time ultrasound during internal jugular cannulation when performed by "properly trained clinicians" and recognize the usefulness of non-real time ultrasound for identification of vessel anatomy and marking optimal skin entry point. Evidence supporting the use of real time ultrasound for subclavian vein cannulation is less clear; however, an overview of the anatomy and sonoanatomy of this area is worthy of review.

SUMMARY

The availability and use of ultrasonography in anesthesia is increasing in parallel with a diversity of indications for its use as technology improves. The clinical application of ultrasonography for the anesthesiologist practicing in the ENT field is in its infancy. This review of published literature shows that ultrasonography has the potential to increase the sensitivity and specificity for prediction of difficult airway, with promising evidence that failure to identify the hyoid bone with sublingual ultrasonography is predictive of a laryngoscopic view of III or greater. The use of ultrasonography to aid the diagnosis of epiglottitis may also prove to be clinically valuable in the management of this acute airway condition, and measurement of air column width to predict occurrence of postextubation stridor has obvious clinical appeal. There is great promise in using ultrasonography to aid safe placement of percutaneous tracheostomy, and location of the cricothyroid membrane and hyoid bone may be of value to assist anesthesia of the airway prior to awake fiberoptic intubation. There is also the possibility for improving success and safety of regional anesthesia of the head and neck through accurate needle placement and injection of local anesthetic. Although the potential for ultrasonography to improve clinical practice seems promising, the full extent of this will only become apparent over time.

Despite the potential for the use of ultrasonography in ENT, many ultrasound approaches described in this review are of academic interest and are not currently practical for routine use by the majority of practicing anesthesiologists or intensivists. Moreover, mastering the technical skills required to successfully interpret and use ultrasonography requires time and a detailed knowledge of the relevant anatomy. Further clinical studies are required to improve our understanding of this subject and to determine whether potential can be converted into tangible clinical benefit.

ACKNOWLEDGMENTS

The authors would like to thank Dr Derek Dillane (Assistant Professor) and Jennifer Pillay (Research Assistant), Department of Anesthesiology and Pain Medicine, University of Alberta, Edmonton, Alberta, Canada for their contributions, as well as Pillay's volunteering as a model for the ultrasound images and photographs. They also thank Jenkin Tsui (Student, Edmonton, Alberta, Canada) for creating the illustrations provided to highlight the relevant regional anatomy of the imaging approaches.

REFERENCES

1. Gray AT. Ultrasound-guided regional anesthesia: current state of the art. Anesthesiology 2006; 104(2):368–73.
2. Soeding P, Eizenberg N. Review article: anatomical considerations for ultrasound guidance for regional anesthesia of the neck and upper limb. Can J Anaesth 2009;56(7):518–33.
3. Singh M, Chin KJ, Chan VW, et al. Use of sonography for airway assessment: an observational study. J Ultrasound Med 2010;29(1):79–85.
4. Bertram S, Emshoff R, Norer B. Ultrasonographic anatomy of the anterior neck: implications for tracheostomy. J Oral Maxillofac Surg 1995;53(12):1420–4.
5. Hatfield A, Bodenham A. Portable ultrasonic scanning of the anterior neck before percutaneous dilatational tracheostomy. Anaesthesia 1999;54(7):660–3.
6. Sustic A, Kovac D, Zgaljardic Z, et al. Ultrasound-guided percutaneous dilatational tracheostomy: a safe method to avoid cranial misplacement of the tracheostomy tube. Intensive Care Med 2000; 26(9):1379–81.
7. Sustic A, Zupan Z. Ultrasound guided tracheal puncture for non-surgical tracheostomy. Intensive Care Med 1998;24(1):92.
8. Sustic A, Zupan Z, Eskinja N, et al. Ultrasonographically guided percutaneous dilatational tracheostomy after anterior cervical spine fixation. Acta Anaesthesiol Scand 1999;43(10):1078–80.
9. Sustic A, Zupan Z, Antoncic I. Ultrasound-guided percutaneous dilatational tracheostomy with laryngeal mask airway control in a morbidly obese patient. J Clin Anesth 2004;16(2):121–3.
10. NAP 4. Available at: http://www.rcoa.ac.uk/. Accessed December 8, 2011.
11. Tsui BC, Tsui J. Rapid percutaneous tracheal catheterization using electrical guidance. Can J Anesth 2012;59(1):116–7.
12. Tsui BC, Hui CM. Challenges in sublingual airway ultrasound interpretation. Can J Anaesth 2009; 56(5):393–4.
13. Prasad A, Singh M, Chan VW. Ultrasound imaging of the airway. Can J Anaesth 2009;56(11):868–9.
14. Werner SL, Jones RA, Emerman CL. Sonographic assessment of the epiglottis. Acad Emerg Med 2004;11(12):1358–60.
15. Garel C, Contencin P, Polonovski JM, et al. Laryngeal ultrasonography in infants and children: a new way of investigating. Normal and pathological findings. Int J Pediatr Otorhinolaryngol 1992;23(2): 107–15.
16. Bektas F, Soyuncu S, Yigit O, et al. Sonographic diagnosis of epiglottal enlargement. Emerg Med J 2010;27(3):224–5.
17. Garel C, Hassan M, Legrand I, et al. Laryngeal ultrasonography in infants and children: pathological findings. Pediatr Radiol 1991;21(3):164–7.
18. Ezri T, Gewurtz G, Sessler DI, et al. Prediction of difficult laryngoscopy in obese patients by ultrasound quantification of anterior neck soft tissue. Anaesthesia 2003;58(11):1111–4.
19. Komatsu R, Sengupta P, Wadhwa A, et al. Ultrasound quantification of anterior soft tissue thickness fails to predict difficult laryngoscopy in obese patients. Anaesth Intensive Care 2007;35(1):32–7.
20. Hui C, Tsui BC. Sublingual ultrasound examination of the airway: a pilot study [abstract 613888]. Canadian Anesthesiologists' Society Annual Meeting 2009. Vancouver, June 26–30, 2009. Available at: http://cas.staging.swiftkicx.com/annual_meeting/abstracts_and_refresher/oral_competition08/pdfs/613888.pdf. Accessed July 21, 2010.
21. Chou HC, Wu TL. Mandibulohyoid distance in difficult laryngoscopy. Br J Anaesth 1993;71(3):335–9.
22. Chou HC, Wu TL. Rethinking the three axes alignment theory for direct laryngoscopy. Acta Anaesthesiol Scand 2001;45(2):261–2.
23. Sustic A. Role of ultrasound in the airway management of critically ill patients. Crit Care Med 2007; 35(Suppl 5):S173–7.
24. Hatfield A, Bodenham A. Ultrasound: an emerging role in anaesthesia and intensive care. Br J Anaesth 1999;83(5):789–800.
25. Raphael DT, Conard FU III. Ultrasound confirmation of endotracheal tube placement. J Clin Ultrasound 1987;15(7):459–62.
26. Werner SL, Smith CE, Goldstein JR, et al. Pilot study to evaluate the accuracy of ultrasonography in confirming endotracheal tube placement. Ann Emerg Med 2007;49(1):75–80.

27. Marciniak B, Fayoux P, Hebrard A, et al. Airway management in children: ultrasonography assessment of tracheal intubation in real time? Anesth Analg 2009;108(2):461–5.

28. Ma G, Davis DP, Schmitt J, et al. The sensitivity and specificity of transcricothyroid ultrasonography to confirm endotracheal tube placement in a cadaver model. J Emerg Med 2007;32(4):405–7.

29. Milling TJ, Jones M, Khan T, et al. Transtracheal 2-D ultrasound for identification of esophageal intubation. J Emerg Med 2007;32(4):409–14.

30. Sustic A, Miletic D, Protic A, et al. Can ultrasound be useful for predicting the size of a left double-lumen bronchial tube? Tracheal width as measured by ultrasonography versus computed tomography. J Clin Anesth 2008;20(4):247–52.

31. Ding LW, Wang HC, Wu HD, et al. Laryngeal ultrasound: a useful method in predicting post-extubation stridor. A pilot study. Eur Respir J 2006;27(2): 384–9.

32. Bohme G. [Ultrasound diagnosis of the epiglottis]. HNO 1990;38(10):355–60 [in German].

33. Wakamatsu T, Tsushima K, Yasuo M, et al. Usefulness of preoperative endobronchial ultrasound for airway invasion around the trachea: esophageal cancer and thyroid cancer. Respiration 2006;73(5): 651–7.

34. Murgu S, Kurimoto N, Colt H. Endobronchial ultrasound morphology of expiratory central airway collapse. Respirology 2008;13(2):315–9.

35. Shaw TJ, Wakely SL, Peebles CR, et al. Endobronchial ultrasound to assess airway wall thickening: validation in vitro and in vivo. Eur Respir J 2004; 23(6):813–7.

36. Deveze A, Sebag F, Hubbard J, et al. Identification of patients with a non-recurrent inferior laryngeal nerve by duplex ultrasound of the brachiocephalic artery. Surg Radiol Anat 2003;25(3-4):263–9.

37. Huang SM, Wu TJ. Neck ultrasound for prediction of right nonrecurrent laryngeal nerve. Head Neck 2010;32(7):844–9.

38. Ooi LL. B-mode real-time ultrasound assessment of vocal cord function in recurrent laryngeal nerve palsy. Ann Acad Med Singap 1992;21(2):214–6.

39. Ooi LL, Chan HS, Soo KC. Color Doppler imaging for vocal cord palsy. Head Neck 1995;17(1):20–3.

40. Sandeman DJ, Griffiths MJ, Lennox AF. Ultrasound guided deep cervical plexus block. Anaesth Intensive Care 2006;34(2):240–4.

41. Usui Y, Kobayashi T, Kakinuma H, et al. An anatomical basis for blocking of the deep cervical plexus and cervical sympathetic tract using an ultrasound-guided technique. Anesth Analg 2010; 110(3):964–8.

42. Kefalianakis F, Koeppel T, Geldner G, et al. [Carotid-surgery in ultrasound-guided anesthesia of the regio colli lateralis]. Anasthesiol Intensivmed Notfallmed Schmerzther 2005;40(10):576–81 [in German].

43. Roessel T, Wiessner D, Heller AR, et al. High-resolution ultrasound-guided high interscalene plexus block for carotid endarterectomy. Reg Anesth Pain Med 2007;32(3):247–53.

44. Tsui BC, Dillane D. Finucane. Neural blockade for surgery to the neck and head: clinical applications. In: Cousins MJ, Bridenbaugh PO, Carr D, et al, editors. Cousin and Bridenbaugh's neural blockade in clinical anesthesia and management of pain. 4th edition. Philadelphia: Lippincott Williams and Wilkins; 2008.

45. Furlan JC. Anatomical study applied to anesthetic block technique of the superior laryngeal nerve. Acta Anaesthesiol Scand 2002;46(2):199–202.

46. Kundra P, Kutralam S, Ravishankar M. Local anaesthesia for awake fibreoptic nasotracheal intubation. Acta Anaesthesiol Scand 2000;44(5):511–6.

47. Reasoner DK, Warner DS, Todd MM, et al. A comparison of anesthetic techniques for awake intubation in neurosurgical patients. J Neurosurg Anesthesiol 1995;7(2):94–9.

48. Hannan L, Reader A, Nist R, et al. The use of ultrasound for guiding needle placement for inferior alveolar nerve blocks. Oral Surg Oral Med Oral Pathol Oral Radiol Endod 1999;87(6):658–65.

49. Pascal J, Charier D, Perret D, et al. Peripheral blocks of trigeminal nerve for facial soft-tissue surgery: learning from failures. Eur J Anaesthesiol 2005; 22(6):480–2.

50. Prabhu KP, Wig J, Grewal S. Bilateral infraorbital nerve block is superior to peri-incisional infiltration for analgesia after repair of cleft lip. Scand J Plast Reconstr Surg Hand Surg 1999;33(1):83–7.

51. Tsui BC. Ultrasound imaging to localize foramina for superficial trigeminal nerve block. Can J Anaesth 2009;56(9):704–6.

52. Greher M, Moriggl B, Curatolo M, et al. Sonographic visualization and ultrasound-guided blockade of the greater occipital nerve: a comparison of two selective techniques confirmed by anatomical dissection. Br J Anaesth 2010;104(5):637–42.

53. Troianos CA, Hartman GS, Glas KE, et al. Councils on Intraoperative Echocardiography and Vascular Ultrasound of the American Society of Echocardiography. Special articles: guidelines for performing ultrasound guided vascular cannulation: recommendations of the American Society of Echocardiography and the Society Of Cardiovascular Anesthesiologists. Anesth Analg 2012;114(1):46–72.

Special Article in Emergengy Ultrasound

The RUSH Exam 2012: Rapid Ultrasound in Shock in the Evaluation of the Critically Ill Patient

Phillips Perera, MD, RDMS[a],*, Thomas Mailhot, MD, RDMS[a],
David Riley, MD, MS, RDMS, RDCS, RVT[b], Diku Mandavia, MD, FRCPC[a]

KEYWORDS
- Rapid ultrasound in shock examination • RUSH exam
- Shock • Ultrasound

Care of the patient with shock can be one of the most challenging issues in Emergency Medicine and Critical Care. Even the most seasoned clinician, standing at the bedside of the patient in extremis, can be unclear about the cause of shock and the optimal initial therapeutic approach. Traditional physical examination techniques can be misleading given the complex physiology of shock.[1] Patients in shock have high mortality rates, and these rates are correlated to the amount and duration of hypotension. Therefore, diagnosis and initial care must be accurate and prompt to optimize patient outcomes.[2] Failure to make the correct diagnosis and act appropriately can lead to potentially disastrous outcomes and a high-risk situation for the provider.

Ultrasound technology has been rapidly integrated into General Medicine and specifically, Emergency Department care, in the last decade. More practicing Emergency Physicians (EP's) and Critical Care Physicians are now trained in bedside point of care, or goal directed, ultrasound and this training is now both supported by the American Medical Association and included in the formal curriculum of all United States Emergency Medicine Residency Programs under the current guidelines from the Accreditation Council for Graduate Medical Education.[3–5] Furthermore, the American College of Emergency Physicians (ACEP) and the Council of Emergency Medicine Residency Directors (CORD) have formally endorsed bedside ultrasound by the EP for multiple applications.[6,7] This technology is ideal for the care of the critical patient in shock, and the most recent ACEP guidelines further delineate a new category of 'resuscitative' ultrasound.[8]

Over the last years, in addition to the original RUSH protocol published in 2010, there have been a number of new resuscitation ultrasound protocols developed to more accurately diagnose the patient in shock and to more rapidly develop an improved care plan in the initial stages of medical care.[1,9–21] Clinicians have also expanded these resuscitation protocols to encompass the ultrasound evaluation of the patient presenting with unexplained dyspnea, incorporating many of the same exam components utilized in the evaluation of shock.[22–25] Instead of relying on older techniques, like listening for changes in sound coming from the patient's body suggestive of specific

This article was previously published in the February 2010 issue of *Emergency Medicine Clinics*. This version represents an update to the original article.
a Department of Emergency Medicine, Los Angeles County+USC Medical Center, General Hospital, 1200 State Street, Room 1011, Los Angeles, CA 90033, USA
b Division of Emergency Medicine, New York Presbyterian Hospital, Columbia University Medical Center, 622 West 168th Street, New York, NY 10032, USA
* Corresponding author.
E-mail address: pperera1@mac.com

pathology, bedside ultrasound now allows direct visualization of both pathology and abnormal physiological states. Thus, in 2012 there is currently a fundamental paradigm shift away from the traditional use of bedside ultrasound focused only on the assessment of patient anatomy toward the use of ultrasound to assess critical patient physiology, making it an essential component in the evaluation of the patient in shock.

CLASSIFICATIONS OF SHOCK

Many authorities categorize shock into 4 classic subtypes.[26] The first is hypovolemic shock. This condition is commonly encountered in the patient who is hemorrhaging from trauma, or from a non-traumatic source of brisk bleeding such as from the gastrointestinal (GI) tract or a rupturing aortic aneurysm. Hypovolemic shock may also result from nonhemorrhagic conditions with extensive loss of body fluids, such as GI fluid loss from vomiting and diarrhea. The second subtype of shock is distributive shock. The classic example of this class of shock is sepsis, in which the vascular system is vasodilated to the point that the core vascular blood volume is insufficient to maintain end organ perfusion. Other examples of distributive shock include neurogenic shock, caused by a spinal cord injury, and anaphylactic shock, a severe form of allergic response. The third major form of shock is cardiogenic shock, resulting from pump failure and the inability of the heart to propel the needed oxygenated blood forward to vital organs. Cardiogenic shock can be seen in patients with advanced cardiomyopathy, myocardial infarction, or acute valvular failure. The last type of shock is obstructive shock. This type is most commonly caused by cardiac tamponade, tension pneumothorax, or large pulmonary embolus. Many patients with obstructive shock will need an acute intervention, such as pericardiocentesis, tube thoracostomy or anticoagulation and possible fibrinolysis.

At the bedside of a critical patient, it is often difficult to assess clinically which classification of shock best fits the patient's current clinical status. Physical findings often overlap between the subtypes. For example, patients with tamponade, cardiogenic shock and sepsis (when myocardial depression compounds this form of distributive shock) may all present with distended neck veins and respiratory distress. Because of this diagnostic challenge, practitioners used to perform Swan-Ganz catheterization in hypotensive patients, providing immediate intravascular hemodynamic data. Although the data obtained from these catheters was detailed and often helpful at the bedside, large studies demonstrated no improvement in mortality in the patients who received such prolonged invasive monitoring.[27] Swan-Ganz catheterization has thus declined in use, and the stage has now been set for development of a noninvasive hemodynamic assessment using point of care ultrasound.

SHOCK ULTRASOUND PROTOCOL: THE RUSH EXAM

Given the advantages of early integration of bedside ultrasound into the diagnostic workup of the patient in shock, this article outlines an easily learned and quickly performed 3-step shock ultrasound protocol. The authors term this new ultrasound protocol the RUSH exam (Rapid Ultrasound in SHock). This protocol involves a 3-part bedside physiologic assessment simplified as:

Step 1: The pump
Step 2: The tank
Step 3: The pipes

This examination is performed using standard ultrasound equipment present in many emergency departments today. The authors recommend a phased-array transducer (3.5–5 MHz) to allow adequate thoracoabdominal intercostal scanning, and a linear array transducer (7.5–10 MHz) for the required venous examinations and for the evaluation of pneumothorax.

The first, and most crucial, step in evaluation of the patient in shock is determination of cardiac status, termed for simplicity "the pump" (**Table 1**). Clinicians caring for the patient in shock begin with a limited echocardiogram. The echo examination is focused on looking for 3 main findings. First, the pericardial sac can be visualized to determine if the patient has a pericardial effusion that may be compressing the heart, leading to a mechanical cause of obstructive shock. Second, the left ventricle can be analyzed for global contractility. Determination of the size and contractility status of the left ventricle will allow for those patients with a cardiogenic cause of shock to be rapidly identified.[28,29] The third goal-directed examination of the heart focuses on determining the relative size of the left ventricle to the right ventricle. A heart that has an increased size of the right ventricle relative to the left ventricle may be a sign of acute right ventricular strain from a massive pulmonary embolus in the hypotensive patient.[30–32]

The second part of the RUSH shock ultrasound protocol focuses on the determination of effective intravascular volume status, which will be referred

Table 1
Rapid Ultrasound in SHock (RUSH) protocol: ultrasonographic findings seen with classic shock states

RUSH Evaluation	Hypovolemic Shock	Cardiogenic Shock	Obstructive Shock	Distributive Shock
Pump	Hypercontractile heart Small chamber size	Hypocontractile heart Dilated heart	Hypercontractile heart Pericardial effusion Cardiac tamponade RV Strain Cardiac thrombus	Hypercontractile heart (early sepsis) Hypocontractile heart (late sepsis)
Tank	Flat IVC Flat jugular veins Peritoneal fluid (fluid loss) Pleural fluid (fluid loss)	Distended IVC Distended jugular veins Lung rockets (pulmonary edema) Pleural fluid (effusions) Peritoneal fluid (ascites)	Distended IVC Distended jugular veins Absent lung sliding (pneumothorax)	Normal or small IVC (early sepsis) Peritoneal fluid (peritonitis) Pleural fluid (empyema)
Pipes	Abdominal aneurysm Aortic dissection	Normal	DVT	Normal

Abbreviations: DVT, deep venous thrombosis; IVC, inferior vena cava; RV, right ventricle.

to as "the tank." Placement of the probe in the subxiphoid position, along both the long and short axis of the inferior vena cava (IVC), will allow correct determination of the size of the vessel. Looking at the respiratory dynamics of the IVC will provide an assessment of the patient's volume status to answer the clinical question, "how full is the tank?"[33–38] The clinician can also place a transducer on the internal jugular veins to view their size and changes in diameter with breathing to further assess volume.[39,40] Also included in evaluation of the tank is an assessment of the lung, pleural cavity, and abdominal cavities for pathology that could signal a compromised vascular volume. Integration of lung ultrasound techniques can quickly allow the clinician to identify a pneumothorax, which in the hypotensive patient may represent a tension pneumothorax requiring immediate decompression. Tension pneumothorax presumably limits venous return into the heart due to increased pressure within the chest cavity.[41,42] The lung can also be examined for ultrasonic B lines, a potential sign of volume overload and pulmonary edema.[43,44] The clinician can further examine the thoracic cavity for a pleural effusion. Last, the clinician can perform a FAST exam (Focused Assessment with Sonography in Trauma), to look for fluid in the abdomen, indicating a source for "loss of fluid from the tank."

The third and final part of the shock ultrasound protocol is evaluation of the large arteries and veins of the body, referred to as "the pipes." Clinicians should answer the clinical question "are the pipes ruptured or obstructed?" by first evaluating the arterial side of the vascular system to specifically examine the abdominal and thoracic aorta for an aneurysm or dissection. Next the clinician should turn to evaluation of the venous side of the vascular system. The femoral and popliteal veins can be examined with a high frequency linear array transducer for compressibility. Lack of full venous compression with direct pressure is highly suggestive of a deep venous thrombosis (DVT).[45–47] Presence of a venous thrombus in the hypotensive patient may signal a large pulmonary thromboembolus.

RUSH Protocol: Step 1—Evaluation of the Pump

Focused echocardiography is a skill that is readily learned by the EP and the use of this application has been supported by a recent consensus document developed by colleagues in Emergency Medicine and Cardiology.[48] Imaging of the heart usually involves 4 views. The traditional views of the heart for bedside echocardiography are the parasternal long and short-axis views, the subxiphoid view and the apical 4-chamber view (**Fig. 1**). The parasternal views are taken with the probe positioned just left of the sternum at intercostal space 3 or 4. The subxiphoid 4-chamber view is obtained with the probe aimed up toward

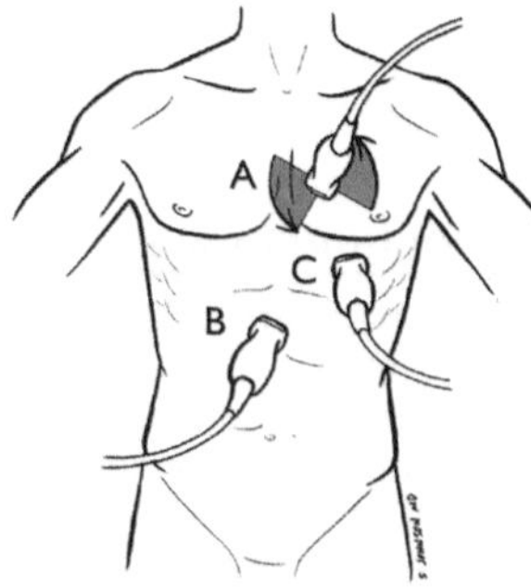

A) Parasternal Views
    Long / Short Axis

B) Subxiphoid View

C) Apical View

Fig. 1. *Rapid Ultrasound in SHock* (RUSH) step 1. Evaluation of the pump.

the left shoulder from a position just below the subxiphoid tip of the sternum (**Fig. 2**). The apical 4-chamber view of the heart is best evaluated by turning the patient into a left lateral decubitus position and placing the probe just below the nipple line at the point of maximal impulse of the heart. It is important for the EP to know all 4 views of the heart, as some views may not be well seen in individual patients, and an alternative view may be needed to answer the clinical question at hand.

"Effusion around the pump": evaluation of the pericardium

The first priority is to search for the presence of a pericardial effusion, which may be a cause of the patient's hemodynamic instability. The heart should be imaged in the planes described here, with close attention to the presence of fluid, usually appearing as a dark or anechoic area, within the pericardial space (**Fig. 3**). Small effusions may be seen as a thin stripe inside the pericardial space, whereas larger effusions tend to

wrap circumferentially around the heart.[49,50] Isolated small anterior anechoic areas on the parasternal long-axis view often represent a pericardial fat pad, as free flowing pericardial effusions will tend to layer posteriorly and inferiorly with gravity. Fresh fluid or blood tends to have a darker or anechoic appearance, whereas clotted blood or exudates may have a lighter or more echogenic look.

Pericardial effusions can result in hemodynamic instability, due to increased pressure within the sac leading to compression of the heart. Because the pericardium is a relatively thick and fibrous structure, acute pericardial effusions may result in cardiac tamponade despite only small amounts of fluid. In contrast, chronic effusions can grow to a large volume without hemodynamic instability.[51] Once a pericardial effusion is identified, the next step is to evaluate the heart for signs of tamponade. Thinking of the heart as a dual chamber in-line pump, the left side of the heart is under considerably more pressure, due to the high systemic pressures against which it must pump. The right side of the heart is under relatively less pressure, due to the lower pressure within the pulmonary vascular circuit. Thus, most echocardiographers define tamponade as compression of the right side of the heart (**Fig. 4**). High pressure within the pericardial sac keeps the chamber from fully expanding during the relaxation phase of the cardiac cycle and thus is best recognized during diastole. As either chamber may be affected by the effusion, both the right atrium and right ventricle should be closely inspected for diastolic collapse. Diastolic collapse of the right atrium or right ventricle appears as a spectrum from a subtle inward serpentine deflection of the outer wall to

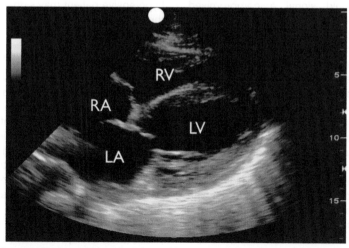

Fig. 2. Subxiphoid view: cardiomyopathy with enlarged heart. LA, left atrium; LV, left ventricle; RA, right atrium; RV, right ventricle.

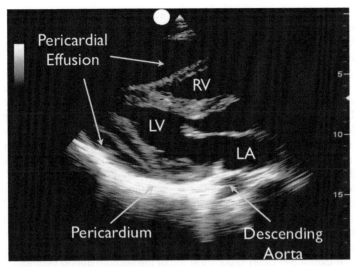

Fig. 3. Parasternal long-axis view: large pericardial effusion.

complete compression of a chamber.[52] Whereas most pericardial effusions are free flowing in the pericardial sac, occasionally effusions may be loculated. This phenomenon is more commonly seen in patients following heart surgery, in whom a clot can form in only one area of the sac.[53] In these cases, effusions can preferentially form posteriorly, and in tamponade, the left side of the heart may be compressed before the right side of the heart. The IVC can also be evaluated for additional confirmatory signs of tamponade.[54,55] IVC plethora will be recognized by distention of the IVC without normal respiratory changes and supports the diagnosis of tamponade (see later discussion of IVC in section "Evaluation of the tank").

Previous published studies have demonstrated that EPs, with a limited amount of training, can correctly and accurately identify the presence of a pericardial effusion.[56] Studies examining the incidence of pericardial effusions in Emergency Department or Intensive Care patients suffering acute shortness of breath, respiratory failure, or shock have found effusions in as many as 13% of these patients.[49] Another study looked specifically at patients arriving at the Emergency Department in near-cardiac arrest states, and found a relatively large number of these cases had pericardial effusions.[57] Thus, symptomatic pericardial effusions may be a cause of hemodynamic instability in a significant number of acute patients,

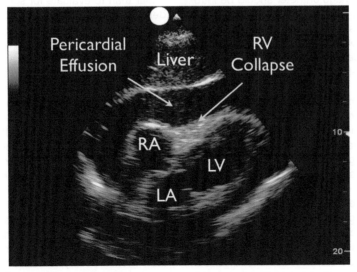

Fig. 4. Subxiphoid view: cardiac tamponade.

and EPs can quickly and accurately diagnose this condition using bedside ultrasound.

As a general principle, it is easier for an EP to diagnose a pericardial effusion than to evaluate for the specific signs of tamponade.[58] It is thus safer to assume tamponade physiology in the hypotensive patient if a significant pericardial effusion is identified. Under ideal circumstances, the EP can obtain a formal echocardiogram in conjunction with Cardiology to specifically examine for cardiac tamponade. In the rare cases where there is not enough time for consultation and the patient is unstable, a pericardiocentesis under ultrasound guidance by the EP may be life-saving. In these cases, employing bedside echocardiography also allows the EP to determine the optimal needle insertion site for pericardiocentesis. Of note, most EPs have classically been taught the subxiphoid approach for pericardiocentesis. However, a large review from the Mayo Clinic looked at 1127 pericardiocentesis procedures, and found that the optimal placement of the needle was where the distance to the effusion was the least and the effusion size was maximal.[59] The apical position at the point of maximal impulse on the left lateral chest wall was chosen in 80% of these procedures, based on these variables. The subxiphoid approach was only chosen in 20% of these procedures, as the investigators recognized the large distance the needle had to travel through the liver to enter the pericardial sac. EPs should therefore anatomically map out the effusion before a pericardiocentesis procedure to plan the most direct and safest route. If the apical approach is selected, the patient should optimally be rolled into a left lateral decubitus position to bring the heart closer to the chest wall, and after local anesthesia, a pericardiocentesis drainage catheter should be introduced over the rib and into the pericardial sac. To maximize success and to avoid complications, the transducer should be placed in a sterile sleeve adjacent to the needle, and the procedure performed under real-time ultrasound guidance.

"Squeeze of the pump": determination of global left ventricular function

The next step in the RUSH protocol is to evaluate the heart for contractility of the left ventricle. This assessment will give a determination of "how strong the pump is." The examination focuses on evaluating motion of the left ventricular endocardial walls, as judged by a visual calculation of the percentage change from diastole to systole. Whereas in the past echocardiographers used radionuclide imaging to determine ejection fraction, published studies have demonstrated that visual determination of contractility is roughly

equivalent.[60] A ventricle that has good contractility will be observed to have a large percentage change from the 2 cycles, with the walls almost coming together and touching during systole. As an example, a vigorously contracting ventricle will almost completely obliterate the ventricular cavity during systole. In comparison, a poorly contracting heart will have a small percentage change in the movement of the walls between diastole and systole. In these hearts, the walls will be observed to move little during the cardiac cycle, and the heart may also be dilated in size, especially if a long-standing cardiomyopathy with severe systolic dysfunction is present. Motion of the anterior leaflet of the mitral valve can also be used to assess contractility. In a normal contractile state, the anterior leaflet will vigorously touch the wall of the septum during ventricular filling when examined using the parasternal long-axis view. M-mode Doppler ultrasound can be used to further document both the motion of the cardiac walls during systole, as well as the movements of the mitral valve leaflets, to better confirm contractility.

The parasternal long-axis view of the heart is an excellent starting view to assess ventricular contractility. Moving the probe into the parasternal short-axis orientation will give confirmatory data on the strength of contractions. In this view, a left ventricle with good contraction will appear as a muscular ring that squeezes down concentrically during systole. Whereas Cardiologists often use the parasternal short-axis view to evaluate for segmental wall motion abnormalities, this is a more subjective measurement, and determinations may differ among different clinicians. For that reason, it is better for the EP to initially concentrate on the overall contractility of the ventricle, rather than to evaluate for segmental wall motion deficits. An easy system of grading is to judge the strength of contractions as good, with the walls of the ventricle contracting well during systole; poor, with the endocardial walls changing little in position from diastole to systole; and intermediate, with the walls moving with a percentage change in between the previous 2 categories. If the parasternal views are inadequate for these determinations, moving the patient into the left lateral decubitus position and examining from the apical view often gives crucial data on left ventricular contractility. The subxiphoid view can be used for this determination, but the left ventricle is farther away from the probe in this view.

Published studies confirm that EP's can perform this examination and get an estimate of left ventricular contractility that compares well with that measured by a Cardiologist.[61] Because a substantial proportion of patients in shock may have a cardiac component to their condition, this part of the examination is very high yield for the clinician.[28] Especially in cases of suspected cardiac ischemia, immediate identification of cardiogenic shock by the EP can lead to more rapid transfer of the patient to the cardiac catheterization suite for revascularization, with a potentially improved outcome.[62,63] Other types of shock can be evaluated by knowing the strength of the left ventricle during systole. Strong ventricular contractility (often termed hyperdynamic, because of the strength of contractions of the left ventricle in addition to a rapid heart rate) is often seen in early sepsis and in hypovolemic shock.[64] In severe hypovolemic conditions, the heart is often small in size with complete obliteration of the ventricular cavity during systole. Bedside echocardiography also allows for repeated evaluation of the patient's heart, looking for changes in contractility over time, especially in the situation when there is an acute deterioration in the patient's status. For example, later in the course of sepsis there may be a decrease in contractility of the left ventricle due to myocardial depression.[65]

Knowing the strength of left ventricular contractility will give the EP a better idea of how much fluid "the pump" or heart of the patient can handle, before manifesting signs and symptoms of fluid overload. This knowledge will serve as a critical guide for the clinician to determine the amount of fluid that can be safely given to a patient. As an example, in a heart with poor contractility, the threshold for initiation of vasopressor agents for hemodynamic support should be lower. In contrast, sepsis patients have been shown to benefit with aggressive early goal-directed therapy, starting with large amounts of fluids before use of vasopressor medications.[66] Because many Emergency Departments do not currently use the invasive catheter needed to optimally monitor the hemodynamic goals outlined for treatment of sepsis patients, bedside ultrasound gives the clinician a noninvasive means to identify and follow a best management strategy.

In cardiac arrest, the clinician should specifically examine for the presence or absence of cardiac contractions. If contractions are seen, the clinician should look for the coordinated movements of the mitral and aortic valves.[67,68] In this scenario, the absence of coordinated opening of mitral and aortic valves will require chest compressions to maintain cardiac output. Specific ultrasound protocols for use in the setting of cardiac arrest, examining the heart, the lungs and the flow in the carotid artery, have been used clinically and further research is ongoing at this time.[69,70] Furthermore, if after prolonged advanced cardiac life support resuscitation the bedside echocardiogram shows cardiac standstill, it is unlikely that the adult patient will have return of spontaneous circulation.[71,72]

"Strain of the pump": assessment of right ventricular strain

In the normal heart, the left ventricle is larger than the right ventricle. This aspect is predominantly a cause of the muscular hypertrophy that takes place in the myocardium of the left ventricle after birth, with the closure of the ductus arteriosus. The left ventricle is under considerably more stress than the right ventricle, to meet the demands of the higher systemic pressure, and hypertrophy is a normal compensatory mechanism. On bedside echocardiography, the normal ratio of the left to right ventricle is 1:0.6.[73] The optimal cardiac views for determining this ratio of size between the 2 ventricles are the parasternal long and short-axis views and the apical 4-chamber view. The subxiphoid view can be used, but care must be taken to scan through the entire right ventricle, as it is possible to underestimate the true right ventricular size if a measurement is taken off-axis.

Any condition that causes pressure to suddenly increase within the pulmonary vascular circuit will result in acute dilation of the right heart in an effort to maintain forward flow into the pulmonary artery. The classic cause of acute right heart strain is a large central pulmonary embolus. Due to the sudden obstruction of the pulmonary outflow tract by a large pulmonary embolus, the compensatory mechanism of acute right ventricular dilation can be viewed on bedside echocardiography. This process will be manifested by a right ventricular chamber with dimensions equivalent to, or larger than, the adjacent left ventricle (**Fig. 5**).[74] In addition, deflection of the interventricular septum from right to left toward the left ventricle may signal higher pressures within the pulmonary artery.[75] In rare cases, intracardiac thrombus may be seen floating free within the heart (**Fig. 6**).[76] In comparison, a condition that causes a more gradual increase in pulmonary artery pressure over time, such as smaller and recurrent pulmonary emboli, cor pulmonale with predominant right heart strain, or primary pulmonary artery hypertension, will cause both dilation and thickening or hypertrophy of the right ventricular wall.[77] These mechanisms can allow the right ventricle to compensate over time and to adapt to pumping blood against the higher pressures in the pulmonary vascular circuit. Acute right heart strain thus differs from chronic right heart strain in that although both conditions cause dilation of the chamber, the ventricle will

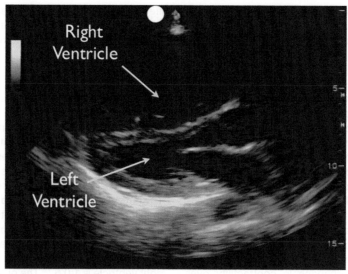

Fig. 5. Parasternal long-axis view: right ventricular strain.

not have the time to hypertrophy if the time course is sudden.

Previous published studies have looked at the sensitivity of the finding of right heart dilation in helping the clinician to diagnose a pulmonary embolus. The results show that the sensitivity is moderate, but the specificity and positive predictive value of this finding are high in the correct clinical scenario, especially if hypotension is present.[30,31,78–80] The presence of acute right heart strain due to a pulmonary embolus correlates with a poorer prognosis.[81,82] This finding, in the setting of suspected pulmonary embolus, suggests the need for immediate evaluation and treatment of thromboembolism.[83] The EP should also proceed directly to evaluation of the leg veins for a DVT (covered in detail later under "Evaluation of the pipes").

The literature suggests that in general, patients with a pulmonary embolus should be immediately started on heparin.[84] However, more recent guidelines, including one from the American Heart Association in 2011, recommend the combined use of anticoagulants and fibrinolytics in the patient with a severe pulmonary embolism, indicated by the presence of hypotension, severe shortness of breath or altered mental status, in the setting of acute right heart strain.[85,86] Bedside, ultrasound gives the treating clinician the clinical confidence to proceed in this more aggressive fashion. Clinical status permitting, a chest computed tomography (CT) scan using

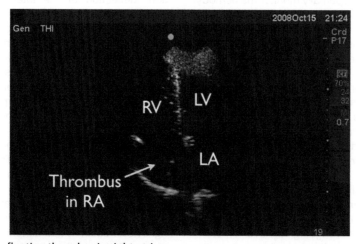

Fig. 6. Apical view: floating thrombus in right atrium.

a dedicated pulmonary embolus protocol should be obtained. If the patient is not stable enough for CT, an emergent echocardiogram in conjunction with Cardiology or bilateral duplex ultrasound of the legs should be considered.

RUSH Protocol Step 2: Evaluation of the Tank

"Fullness of the tank": evaluation of the inferior cava and jugular veins for size and collapse with inspiration

The next step for the clinician using the RUSH protocol in the hypotensive patient is to evaluate the effective intravascular volume as well as to look for areas where the intravascular volume might be compromised (**Fig. 7**). An estimate of the intravascular volume can be determined noninvasively by looking initially at the IVC.[33,34] An effective means of accurately locating and assessing the IVC is to begin with the probe placed in the standard 4-chamber subxiphoid position from the epigastric position, first identifying the right atrium. The probe is then rotated inferiorly toward the spine, examining for the confluence of the IVC with right atrium. The IVC should then be followed inferiorly as it passes through the liver, specifically looking for the convergence of the three hepatic veins with the IVC. Current recommendations for the measurement of the IVC are at the point just inferior to the confluence with the hepatic veins, at a point approximately 2 cm from the junction of right atrium and IVC.[87] Examining the IVC in an oval appearance from the short axis potentially allows the vessel to be more accurately measured, as it avoids a falsely lower measurement by slicing to the side of the vessel, a pitfall known as the cylinder effect. The IVC can also be evaluated in the long-axis plane to further confirm the accuracy of vessel measurements. For this view, the probe is turned from a 4-chamber subxiphoid orientation into a 2-chamber subxiphoid configuration, with the probe now in a vertical orientation and the indicator oriented anteriorly. The aorta will often come first into view from this plane as a thicker walled and pulsatile structure, located deeper to the IVC. Moving the probe toward the patient's right side will then bring the IVC into view. While the IVC may have pulsations, due to its proximity to the aorta, it will often be compressible with direct pressure. Color Doppler ultrasound will also further discriminate the arterial pulsations of the aorta from the phasic movement of blood associated with respirations in the IVC.

As the patient breathes, the IVC will have a normal pattern of collapse during inspiration, due to the negative pressure generated within the chest, causing increased blood flow from the abdominal to the thoracic cavity (**Fig. 8**). This respiratory variation can be further augmented by having the patient sniff, or inspire forcefully. M-Mode Doppler, positioned on the IVC in both short and long-axis planes, can graphically document the dynamic changes in the vessel caliber during the patient's respiratory cycle (**Fig. 9**).

Previous studies have demonstrated a correlation between the size and percentage change of the IVC with respiratory variation to central venous pressure (CVP) using an indwelling catheter. A smaller caliber IVC (<2 cm diameter) with an inspiratory collapse greater than 50% roughly correlates to a CVP of less than 10 mm Hg. This phenomenon may be observed in hypovolemic and distributive shock states. A larger sized IVC (>2 cm diameter) that collapses less than 50% with inspiration correlates to a CVP of more than 10 mm Hg (**Fig. 10**).[88,89] This phenomenon may be seen in cardiogenic and obstructive shock states. New published guidelines by the American Society of Echocardiography support this general use of evaluation of IVC size and collapsibility in assessment of CVP, but suggest more specific ranges for the pressure measurements. The recommendations are that an IVC diameter less than 2.1 cm that collapses greater than 50% with sniff correlates to a normal CVP pressure of 3 mm Hg (range 0-5 mm Hg), while a larger IVC greater than 2.1 cm that collapses less than 50% with sniff suggests a high CVP pressures of 15 mm Hg (range 10-20 mm Hg). In scenarios in which the IVC diameter and collapse do not fit this paradigm, an intermediate value of 8 mm Hg (range 5-10 mm) may be used.[90]

Two caveats to this rule exist. The first is in patients who have received treatment with vasodilators and/or diuretics prior to ultrasound evaluation in whom the IVC may be smaller than prior to treatment, altering the initial physiological state. The second caveat exists in intubated patients

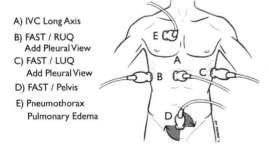

A) IVC Long Axis

B) FAST / RUQ
   Add Pleural View

C) FAST / LUQ
   Add Pleural View

D) FAST / Pelvis

E) Pneumothorax
   Pulmonary Edema

Fig. 7. RUSH step 2. Evaluation of the tank. IVC exam, inferior vena cava; FAST views (Focused Sonography in Trauma), right upper quadrant, left upper quadrant and suprapubic; lung exam, pneumothorax and pulmonary edema.

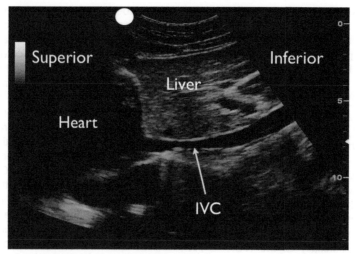

Fig. 8. Inferior vena cava sniff test: low cardiac filling pressures.

receiving positive pressure ventilation, in which the respiratory dynamics of the IVC are reversed. In these patients, the IVC is also less compliant and more distended throughout all respiratory cycles. However, crucial physiologic data can still be obtained in these ventilated patients, as fluid responsiveness has been correlated with an increase in IVC diameter over time.[91]

However, rather than relying on any single measurement of IVC, it may may be more effective to follow the changes in size and respiratory dynamics over time with medical resuscitation, to directly assess real-time changes in patient physiology.[91,92] Observing a change in IVC size from small, with a high degree of inspiratory collapse, to a larger IVC with little respiratory collapse,

following intravenous fluid loading suggests that the CVP is increasing and "the tank" is more full.[93] In contrast, observing a less distended IVC with an increase in respiratory collapse in a patient with a cardiogenic cause of shock following therapy, suggests a decrease in the CVP and a beneficial shift leftward on the Frank-Startling curve to potentiate cardiac output.

The internal jugular veins can also be examined with ultrasound to further evaluate the intravascular volume. As with visual evaluation of the jugular veins, the patient's head is placed at a 30° angle. Using a high-frequency linear array transducer, the internal jugular veins can first be found in the short-axis plane, then evaluated more closely by moving the probe into a long-axis

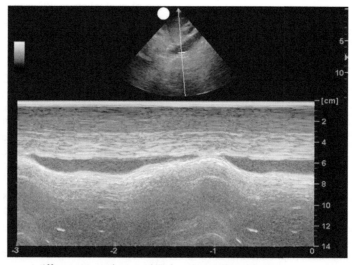

Fig. 9. Inferior vena cava sniff test: M-mode Doppler showing collapsible IVC.

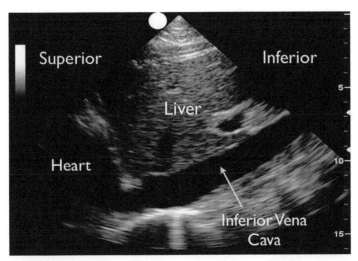

Fig. 10. Inferior vena cava sniff test: high cardiac filling pressures.

configuration. The location of the superior closing meniscus is determined by the point at which the walls of the vein touch each other. Similar to the IVC, the jugular veins can also be examined during respiratory phases to view inspiratory collapse. Veins that are distended, with a closing meniscus level that is high in the course of the neck, suggest a higher CVP.[39,94] Coupling this data with the evaluation of the IVC may give a better overall assessment of the effective intravascular volume. In addition, more advanced Tissue Doppler measurements of the mitral and tricuspid valves, as well as the right ventricular wall, have been proposed as effective means of estimating right atrial pressures and CVP in patients in whom it may be difficult to assess the IVC or jugular veins.[95,96]

"Leakiness of the tank": FAST exam and pleural fluid assessment

Once a patient's intravascular volume status has been determined, the next step in assessing the tank is to look for "abnormal leakiness of the tank." Leakiness of the tank refers to 1 of 3 things leading to hemodynamic compromise: internal blood loss, fluid extravasation, or other pathologic fluid collections. In traumatic conditions, the clinician must quickly determine whether hemoperitoneum or hemothorax is present, as a result of a "hole in the tank," leading to hypovolemic shock. In nontraumatic conditions, accumulation of excess fluid into the abdominal and chest cavities often signifies "tank overload," with resultant pleural effusions and ascites that may build-up with failure of the heart, kidneys, and/or liver. However, many patients with intra-thoracic or intra-abdominal fluid collections may actually be

intravascularly volume depleted, confusing the clinical picture. Focusing on "tank fullness" by assessment of IVC and jugular veins in conjunction with the aforementioned findings can be very helpful in elucidating these conditions. In infectious states, pneumonia may be accompanied by a complicating parapneumonic pleural effusion, and ascites may lead to spontaneous bacterial peritonitis. Depending on the clinical scenario, small fluid collections within the peritoneal cavity may also represent intra-abdominal abscesses leading to a sepsis picture.

The peritoneal cavity can be readily evaluated with bedside ultrasound for the presence of an abnormal fluid collection in both trauma and non-trauma states. This assessment is accomplished with the FAST exam. This examination consists of an inspection of the potential spaces in the right and left upper abdominal quadrants and in the pelvis. Specific views include the space between the liver and kidney (hepatorenal space or Morison's pouch), the area around the spleen (perisplenic space), and the area around and behind the bladder (rectovesicular/rectovaginal space or pouch of Douglas). A dark or anechoic area in any of these 3 potential spaces represents free intraperitoneal fluid (**Fig. 11**). These 3 areas represent the most common places for free fluid to collect, and correspond to the most dependent areas of the peritoneal cavity in the supine patient. Because the FAST exam relies on free fluid settling into these dependent areas, the patient's position should be taken into account while interpreting the examination. Trendelenburg positioning will cause fluid to shift to the upper abdominal regions, whereas an upright position will cause shift of fluid into the pelvis.

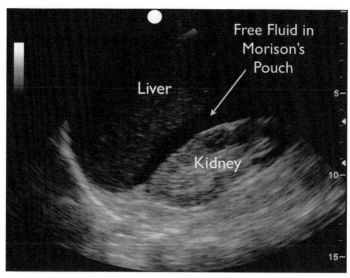

Fig. 11. Right upper quadrant/hepatorenal view: free fluid.

The FAST exam has been reported to detect intraperitoneal fluid collections as small as 100 mL, with a range of 250 to 620 mL commonly cited.[97,98] How much fluid can be detected depends on the clinician's experience as well as the location of the free fluid, with the pelvic view best able to detect small quantities of fluid.[99] The overall sensitivity and specificity of the FAST exam have been reported to be approximately 79% and 99%, respectively.[100,101]

Ultrasound can also assist in evaluating the thoracic cavity for free fluid (pleural effusion or hemothorax) in an examination known as the extended FAST, or E-FAST. This evaluation is easily accomplished by including views of the thoracic cavity with the FAST examination. In both the hepatorenal and perisplenic views, the diaphragms appear as bright or hyperechoic lines immediately above, or cephalad to, the liver and spleen respectively. Aiming the probe above the diaphragm will allow for identification of a thoracic fluid collection. If fluid is found, movement of the probe 1 or 2 intercostal spaces cephalad provides a better view of the thoracic cavity, allowing quantification of the fluid present. In the normal supradiaphragmatic view, there are no dark areas of fluid in the thoracic cavity, and the lung can often be visualized as a moving structure. In the presence of an effusion or hemothorax, the normally visualized lung above the diaphragm is replaced with a dark, or anechoic, space. The lung may also be visualized floating within the pleural fluid (**Fig. 12**). Pleural effusions often exert compression on the lung, causing "hepatization," or an appearance of the lung in the effusion similar to a solid organ, like the liver. The literature supports the use of bedside ultrasound for the detection of pleural effusion and hemothorax. Several studies have found Emergency Department ultrasound to have a sensitivity in excess of 92% and a specificity approaching 100% in the detection of hemothorax.[102–105] Assessing the patient with the head slightly elevated may improve the sensitivity of this examination, as this will cause intrathoracic fluid to accumulate just above the diaphragms.

Free fluid in the peritoneal or thoracic cavities in a hypotensive patient in whom a history of trauma is present or suspected should initially be presumed to be blood, leading to a diagnosis of hemorrhagic shock. Although a history of trauma is commonly elicited in such cases, the trauma may be occult or minor, making diagnosis sometimes difficult. One circumstance of occult trauma is a delayed splenic rupture resulting from an enlarged and more fragile spleen, such as in a patient with infectious mononucleosis. Although rare, this entity may occur several days following a minor trauma, and may thus be easily overlooked by both patient and clinician.[106] Leakage of intestinal contents from rupture of a hollow viscus or urine extravasation from intraperitoneal bladder rupture may also demonstrate free intraperitoneal fluid.

Nontraumatic conditions may also lead to hemorrhagic shock, and must remain on the EP's differential diagnosis. Ruptured ectopic pregnancy and hemorrhagic corpus luteum cyst are 2 diagnoses that should not be overlooked in women of childbearing age. In an elderly patient, an abdominal aortic aneurysm may occasionally rupture into the peritoneal cavity and thoracic aneurysms may rupture into the chest cavity.

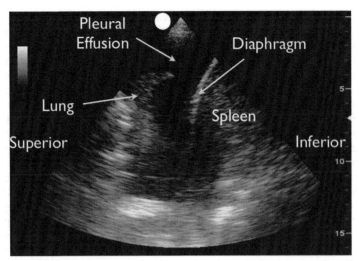

Fig. 12. Left upper quadrant: pleural effusion.

Once the diagnosis of hemorrhagic shock is made, treatment should be directed toward transfusion of blood products and surgical or angiographic intervention.

In the nontrauma patient, ascites and pleural effusions will appear as dark, or anechoic, fluid collections, similar to blood. Parapneumonic inflammation may cause considerable pleural effusions and/or empyema. Differentiating blood from other fluids can be suggested from the history, clinical examination, and chest radiograph. There may occasionally be some signature sonographic findings that help make a diagnosis. In hemorrhagic conditions, blood often has a mixed appearance, with areas of both anechoic fresh blood and more echogenic blood clot present. In an infectious parapneumonic pleural effusion or in spontaneous bacterial peritonitis, the fluid may have a slightly different appearance, with more echogenic debris noted to float in the fluid. Gas bubbles may also be seen in cases of empyema, suggesting an infection within the fluid. Bedside ultrasound can be very helpful in these cases by allowing the clinician to decide if an emergent aspiration of a fluid collection in the chest or abdomen can be safely performed.[107] The results of the fluid aspirated from the patient can then guide further management, as in addition to antibiotics, a more definitive surgical procedure may be indicated to optimize the treatment of the infection.

"Tank compromise": pneumothorax

Although the exact mechanism by which tension pneumothorax causes shock is controversial, it has historically been thought to produce obstructive shock.[41,42,108] According to this theory,

severely increased intrathoracic pressure produces mediastinal shift, which kinks and compresses the inferior and superior vena cava at their insertion into the right atrium, obstructing venous return to the heart. Regardless of the exact mechanism, detection is critical.

Although chest radiography reveals characteristic findings in tension pneumothorax, therapy should not be delayed while awaiting radiographic studies. With bedside ultrasound, the diagnosis of tension pneumothorax can be accomplished within seconds. Pneumothorax detection with ultrasound relies on the fact that free air (pneumothorax) is lighter than normal aerated lung tissue, and thus will accumulate in the nondependent areas of the thoracic cavity. Therefore, in a supine patient a pneumothorax will be found anteriorly, while in an upright patient a pneumothorax will be found superiorly at the lung apex.

Multiple studies have shown ultrasound to be more sensitive than supine chest radiography for the detection of pneumothorax.[109–115] Sensitivities for these various studies ranged from 86% to 100%, with specificities ranging from 92% to 100%. A study by Zhang and colleagues[112] that focused on trauma victims found the sensitivity of ultrasound for pneumothorax was 86% versus 27% for chest radiography; furthermore, this same study reported the average time to obtain ultrasound was 2.3 minutes versus 19.9 minutes for chest radiography.

To assess for pneumothorax with ultrasound, the patient should be positioned in a supine position, or even more optimally, with the head of the bead slightly elevated. By looking at the patient from a lateral orientation, one can assess the most anterior portion of the chest cavity.

Subsequent positioning of a high frequency linear array probe at this highest point on the thorax, usually found in the mid-clavicular line at approximately the second through fourth intercostal positions, allows identification of the pleural line. This line appears as an echogenic horizontal line located approximately half a centimeter deep to the ribs. The pleural line consists of both the visceral and parietal pleura closely apposed to one another. In the normal lung, the visceral and parietal pleura can be seen to slide against each other, with a glistening or shimmering appearance, as the patient breathes (**Fig. 13**). The presence of this lung sliding excludes a pneumothorax.[116] This lung sliding motion can be graphically depicted by using M-mode Doppler. A normal image will depict "waves on the beach," with no motion of the chest wall anteriorly, represented as linear "waves," and the motion of the lung posteriorly, representing "the beach" (**Fig. 14**). When a pneumothorax is present, air gathers between the parietal and visceral pleura, preventing the ultrasound beam from detecting lung sliding. In pneumothorax, the pleural line identified with ultrasound will consist only of the parietal layer, seen as a single stationary line. While the line may be seen to move anteriorly and posteriorly due to exaggerated chest wall motions, especially in cases of severe dyspnea and respiratory distress, the characteristic horizontal respiratory sliding of the pleural line back and forth will not be seen. M-mode Doppler through the chest will show only repeating horizontal linear lines, demonstrating a lack of lung sliding or absence of the "beach" (see **Fig. 14**). Although the presence of lung sliding is sufficient to rule out pneumothorax, the absence of lung sliding may be seen in other conditions in addition to pneumothorax, such as a chronic obstructive pulmonary disease bleb, consolidated pneumonia, atelectasis, or mainstem intubation.[117–119] Thus the absence of lung sliding, especially as defined in one intercostal space, is not by itself diagnostic of a pneumothorax. The clinician can examine through several more intercostal spaces, moving the transducer more inferiorly and lateral, to increase the utility of the test. This maneuver may also help identify the lung point, or the area where an incomplete pneumothorax interfaces with the chest wall, as visualized by the presence of lung sliding on one side and the lack of lung sliding on the other.[120]

Another sonographic finding seen in normal lung, but absent in pneumothorax, is the comet tail artifact. Comet tail artifact is a form of reverberation echo that arises from irregularity of the lung surface. This phenomenon appears as a vertical hyperechoic line originating from the pleural line and extending down into the lung tissue. The presence of comet tail artifact rules out a pneumothorax.[121] The combination of a lack of lung sliding and absent comet tail artifacts strongly suggests pneumothorax. In the setting of undifferentiated shock, the EP should strongly consider that a tension pneumothorax may be present, and immediate needle decompression followed by tube thoracostomy should be considered.

"Tank overload": pulmonary edema
Pulmonary edema often accompanies cardiogenic shock, in which weakened cardiac function causes a backup of blood into the pulmonary vasculature, leading to tank overload. Yet the clinical picture can be misleading, as patients in pulmonary edema may present with wheezing, rather than rales, or may have relatively clear lung sounds. The ability to quickly image the lung fields with ultrasound can rapidly lead the EP to the correct diagnosis. Although it is a relatively new concept, ultrasound has been shown to be helpful in the detection of pulmonary edema.[122,123] The sonographic signs of pulmonary edema correlate well with chest radiography.[124]

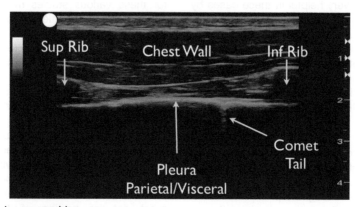

Fig. 13. Long-axis view: normal lung.

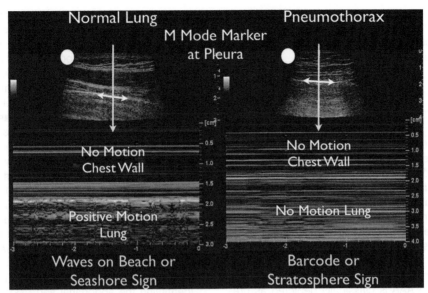

Fig. 14. M-mode: normal lung versus pneumothorax.

To assess for pulmonary edema with ultrasound, the lungs are scanned with the phased-array transducer in the anterolateral chest between the second and fifth rib interspaces. A more recent study has suggested that the lungs should also be examined from a more lateral orientation, or even from a posterior approach, to better increase the sensitivity of this technique in the detection of pulmonary edema.[125] Detection of pulmonary edema with ultrasound relies on seeing a special type of lung ultrasound artifact, termed ultrasound B lines (**Fig. 15**). These B lines appear as a series of diffuse, brightly echogenic lines originating from the pleural line and projecting in a fanlike pattern into the thorax (described as "lung rockets"). In contrast to the smaller comet tail artifacts seen in normal lung that fade out within a few centimeters of the pleural line, the B lines of pulmonary edema are better defined and extend to the far field of the ultrasound image. B lines result from thickening of the interlobular septa, as extravascular water accumulates within the pulmonary interstitium.[122,124] The presence of B lines coupled with decreased cardiac contractility and a plethoric IVC on focused sonographic evaluation should prompt the clinician to consider the presence of pulmonary edema and initiate appropriate treatment. Interestingly, a decrease in the number of B lines noted over time with ultrasound examination of a patient's chest following

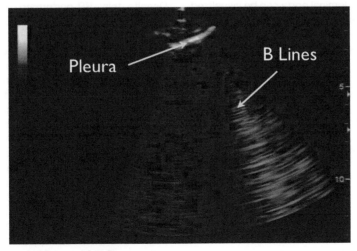

Fig. 15. Lung ultrasound: edema with B lines.

medical treatment has been correlated with an improvement in their clinical condition, secondary to an overall decrease in the absolute amount of water in the lungs.[126]

RUSH Protocol: Step 3—Evaluation of the Pipes

"Rupture of the pipes": aortic aneurysm and dissection

The next step in the RUSH exam is to examine the 'Pipes' looking first at the arterial side of the circulatory system and then at the venous side (**Fig. 16**). Vascular catastrophes, such as ruptured abdominal aortic aneurysms (AAA) and aortic dissections, are life-threatening causes of hypotension. The survival of such patients may often be measured in minutes, and the ability to quickly diagnose these diseases is crucial.

A ruptured AAA is classically depicted as presenting with back pain, hypotension, and a pulsatile abdominal mass. However, fewer than half of cases occur with this triad, and some cases will present with shock as the only finding.[127] A large or rupturing AAA can also mimic a kidney stone, with flank pain and hematuria. Fortunately for the EP, ultrasound can be used to rapidly diagnose both conditions.[128] Numerous studies have shown that EPs can make the diagnosis of AAA using bedside ultrasound, with a high sensitivity and specificity.[129–132] The sensitivity of EP-performed ultrasound for the detection of AAA ranges from 93% to 100%, with specificities approaching 100%.[129–131]

A complete ultrasound examination of the abdominal aorta involves imaging from the epigastrium down to the iliac bifurcation using a phased-array or curvilinear transducer. Aiming the transducer posteriorly in a transverse orientation in the epigastric area, the abdominal aorta can be visualized as a circular vessel seen immediately anterior to

the vertebral body and to the left of the paired IVC. Application of steady pressure to the transducer to displace bowel gas, while sliding the probe inferiorly from a position just below the xiphoid process down to the umbilicus, allows for visualization of the entire abdominal aorta. The aorta should also be imaged in the longitudinal orientation for completion. Measurements should be obtained in the short axis, measuring the maximal diameter of the aorta from outer wall to outer wall, and should include any thrombus present in the vessel. A measurement of greater than 3 cm is abnormal and defines an abdominal aortic aneurysm (**Fig. 17**). Smaller aneurysms may be symptomatic, although rupture is more common with aneurysms measuring larger than 5 cm.[133] Studies have also confirmed that the EP can reliably make a correct determination of the size of an AAA.[130,134]

Identifying the abdominal aorta along its entire course is essential to rule out an aneurysm, paying special attention below the renal arteries where most AAAs are located. Rupture of an abdominal aortic aneurysm typically occurs into the retroperitoneal space, which unfortunately is an area difficult to visualize with ultrasound. In a stable patient, a CT scan with intravenous contrast can be ordered to investigate leakage of an aneurysm. However, a hypotensive patient with sonographic evidence of an AAA should be considered to have acute rupture, and a surgeon should be consulted with plans for immediate transport to the operating room.

Another crucial part of "the pipes" protocol is evaluation for an aortic dissection. The sensitivity of transthoracic echocardiography to detect aortic dissection is poor (approximately 65% according to one study), and is limited compared with CT, MRI, or transesophageal echocardiography.[135] Despite this, EP-performed bedside ultrasound has been used to detect aortic dissections and has helped many patients.[136–139] Sonographic findings suggestive of the diagnosis include the presence of aortic root dilation and an aortic intimal flap. The parasternal long-axis view of the heart permits an evaluation of the proximal aortic root, and a measurement of more than 3.8 cm is considered abnormal. An echogenic intimal flap may be recognized within the dilated root or anywhere along the course of the thoracic or abdominal aorta (**Fig. 18**). The suprasternal view allows imaging of the aortic arch and should be performed in high-suspicion scenarios by placing the phased-array transducer within the suprasternal notch and aiming caudally and anteriorly (**Fig. 19**). Color flow Doppler imaging can further delineate 2 lumens with distinct blood flow,

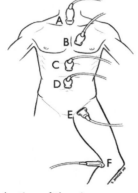

A) Suprasternal Aorta
B) Parasternal Aorta
C) Epigastric Aorta
D) Supraumbilical Aorta
E) Femoral DVT
F) Popliteal DVT

Fig. 16. RUSH step 3. Evaluation of the pipes.

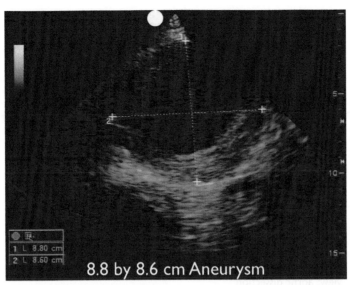

Fig. 17. Short-axis view: large abdominal aortic aneurysm.

confirming the diagnosis. In patients with acute proximal dissection, aortic regurgitation or a pericardial effusion may also be recognized. Abdominal aortic ultrasound may reveal a distal thoracic aortic dissection that extends below the diaphragm, and in the hands of skilled sonographers has been shown to be 98% sensitive.[140]

"Clogging of the pipes": venous thromboembolism
Bedside ultrasound for DVT In the patient in whom a thromboembolic event is suspected as a cause of shock, the EP should then move to an assessment of the venous side of "the pipes." As the majority of pulmonary emboli originate from lower extremity DVT, the examination is concentrated on a limited compression evaluation of the leg veins. Simple compression ultrasonography, which uses a high frequency linear probe to apply direct pressure to the vein, has a good overall sensitivity for detection of DVT of the leg.[141] An acute blood clot forms a mass in the lumen of the vein, and the pathognomonic finding of DVT will be incomplete compression of the anterior and posterior walls of the vein (**Fig. 20**).[142,143] In contrast, a normal vein will completely collapse

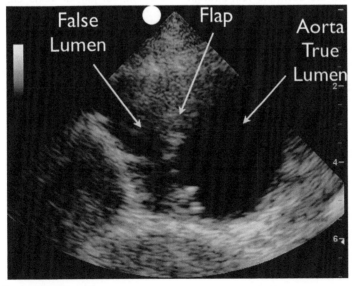

Fig. 18. Short-axis view: aortic dissection.

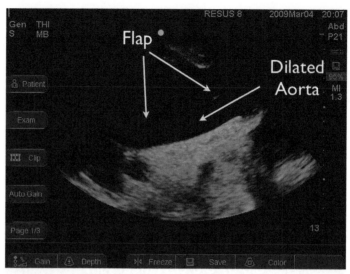

Fig. 19. Suprasternal view: aortic dissection.

with simple compression. Most distal deep venous thromboses can be detected through simple compression ultrasonography of the leg using standard B-mode imaging, and more complicated Doppler techniques add little utility to the examination.[144]

Ultrasound may miss some clots that have formed in the calf veins, a difficult area to evaluate with sonography.[145] However, most proximal DVTs can be detected by a limited compression examination of the leg that can be rapidly performed by focusing on 2 major areas.[146,147] The proximal femoral vein just below the inguinal ligament is evaluated first, beginning at the common femoral vein, found below the inguinal ligament. Scanning should continue down the vein through the confluence with the saphenous vein to the bifurcation of the vessel into the deep and superficial femoral veins. The second area of evaluation is the popliteal fossa. The popliteal vein, the continuation of the superficial femoral vein, can be examined from high in the popliteal fossa down to trifurcation into the calf veins. If an upper extremity thrombus is clinically suspected, the same compression techniques can be employed, following the arm veins up to the axillary vein and into the subclavian vein. While a good initial test, the sensitivity of ultrasound for proximal upper extremity clots is lower than for lower extremity clots, as the subclavian vein cannot be easily compressed behind the clavicle.[148] In addition, the internal jugular veins can be examined for

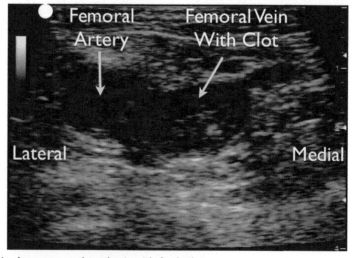

Fig. 20. Femoral vein deep venous thrombosis with fresh clot.

thrombus, a crucial step in assessment for a potential safe location for placement of a central venous catheter, especially if more secure vascular access or administration of vasopressors is needed.

Previous studies have shown that EPs can perform limited ultrasound compression for lower extremity venous clots with good sensitivity in patients with a high pretest probability for the disease.[47,149–152] The examination can also be performed rapidly, and can be integrated into the overall RUSH protocol with a minimum of added time.[153]

SUMMARY

Bedside ultrasound technology has evolved to the point that it offers a powerful, yet easy to use tool for the clinician faced with a critical patient. The initial imaging focus of ultrasound as used by Radiologists was on anatomy and pathology. Now with clinicians actively using this technology at the bedside, attention has shifted to the crucial evaluation of *physiology*. The ability to recognize both abnormal pathology and physiology in a critical patient, recognize a distinctive shock state, and arrive at a more precise diagnosis represents a new paradigm in resuscitation care. Clinicians around the world are recognizing the power of point of care ultrasound and the impact it will have on critical care resuscitation in the Emergency Department, as well as in Intensive Care Units.

The individual components of the *R*apid *U*ltrasound in *SH*ock protocol have been studied and published prior, but this new protocol represents the first synthesis of these sonographic techniques into a unified 3 step algorithm. The protocol simplifies the ultrasound evaluation into the physiological paradigm of "pump, tank, and pipes," allowing the clinician to easily remember the critical aspects of the exam components. Previous criticism of the RUSH exam focusing on the number of ultrasound exam components involved and the potential time taken to perform the entire protocol are not supported by the author's recommendations that individual parts of the exam should be emphasized by the clinical context and that it may not be necessary to complete the entire protocol to gain the valuable information needed to best treat the patient in shock. Unlike previous published studies that have examined ultrasound protocols in the hypotensive patient, the described RUSH exam presents the most detailed shock algorithm for use by EPs to date.[154] By focusing on both the anatomy and the physiology of these complex patients, in shock, bedside ultrasound provides the opportunity for improved clinical treatments and patient outcomes.

For educational videos covering all RUSH applications, please go to http://www.sound-bytes.tv. This site contains a series of free access videos to further teach the clinician how to perform the RUSH exam.

ACKNOWLEDGMENTS

We would like to acknowledge the work of Scott Weingart, MD and Brett Nelson, MD on ultrasound evaluation of the hypotensive patient.

REFERENCES

1. Jones AE, Tayal VS, Sullivan DM, et al. Randomized, controlled trial of immediate versus delayed goal directed ultrasound to identify the cause of nontraumatic hypotension in emergency department patients. Crit Care Med 2004;32:1703–8.
2. Jones AE, Aborn LS, Kline JA. Severity of emergency department hypotension predicts adverse hospital outcome. Shock 2004;22:410–4.
3. Thomas HA, Beeson MS, Binder LS, et al. The 2005 model of the clinical practice of emergency medicine: the 2007 update. Acad Emerg Med 2008; 15(8):776–9.
4. Heller MB, Mandavia D, Tayal VS. Residency training in emergency ultrasound: fulfilling the mandate. Acad Emerg Med 2002;9:835–9.
5. American Medical Association. Amendment H–230.960: Privileging for ultrasound imaging.
6. ACEP emergency ultrasound guidelines. Ann Emerg Med 2009;53:550–70.
7. Akhtar S, Theodoro D, Gaspari R, et al. Resident training in emergency ultrasound: concensus recommendations from the 2008 council of emergency medicine residency directors conference. Acad Emerg Med 2009;16:S32–6.
8. ACEP Policy Statement. Emergency ultrasound imaging criteria compendium. Approved by the ACEP Board of Directors 2006.
9. Perera P, Mailhot T, Riley D, et al. The RUSH exam: Rapid Ultrasound in SHock in the evaluation of the critically ill. Emerg Med Clin N Am 2010;28:29–56.
10. Plummer D, Heegaard W, Dries D, et al. Ultrasound in HEMS: its role in differentiating shock states. Air Med J 2003;22:33–6.
11. Pershad J, Myers S, Plouman C, et al. Bedside limited echocardiography by the emergency physician is accurate during evaluation of the critically ill patient. Pediatrics 2004;114:e667–71.
12. Jensen MB, Sloth E, Larsen M, et al. Transthoracic echocardiography for cardiopulmonary

monitoring in intensive care. Eur J Anaesthesiol 2004;21:700–7.

13. Gunst M, Gaemmaghami V, Sperry J. Accuracy of cardiac function and volume status estimates using the bedside echocardiographic assessment in trauma/critical care. J Trauma 2008;65:509–16.

14. Atkinson PRT, McAuley DJ, Kendall RJ, et al. Abdominal and cardiac evaluation with sonography in shock (ACES): an approach by emergency physicians for use of ultrasound in patients with undifferentiated hypotension. Emerg Med J 2009;26:87–91.

15. Wright J, Jarman R, Connoly J, et al. Echocardiography in the emergency department. Emerg Med J 2009;26:82–6.

16. Elmer J, Noble VA. An evidence based approach for integrating bedside ultrasound into routine practice in the assessment of undifferentiated shock. ICU Director 2010;1(3):163–74.

17. Ferrada P, Murthi S, Anand RJ, et al. Transthoracic focused rapid echocardiography examination: real-time evaluation of fluid status in critically ill trauma patients. J Trauma 2010;70(1):56–64.

18. Grifee MJ, Merkel MJ, Wei KS. The role of echocardiography in hemodynamic assessment of septic shock. Crit Care Clin 2010;26:365–82.

19. Price S, Uddin S, Quinn T. Echocardiography in cardiac arrest. Curr Opin Crit Care 2010;16:211–5.

20. Lanctot YF, Valois M, Bealieu Y. EGLS: echo guided life support. An algorithmic approach to undifferentiated shock. Crit Ultra J 2011;3:123–9.

21. Byrne MW, Hwang JQ. Ultrasound in the critically ill. Ultrasound Clin 2011;6:235–59.

22. Feissel M, Maizel J, Robles G. Clinical relevance of echocardiography in acute severe dyspnea. J Am Society Echocardiogr 2009;22:1159–64.

23. Liteplo AS, Marrill KA, Villen T, et al. Emergency thoracic ultrasound in the differentiation of the etiology of shortness of breath (ETUDES): sonographic B-lines and N-terminal pro-brain-type natriuretic peptide in diagnosing heart failure. Acad Em Med 2009;16:201–10.

24. Cardinale L, Volpicelli G, Binello F, et al. Clinical application of lung ultrasound in patients with acute dyspnea; differential diagnosis between cardiogenic and pulmonary causes. Radiol Med 2009;114:1053–64.

25. Manson W, Hafez NM. The rapid assessment of dyspnea with ultrasound: RADIUS. Ultrasound Clin 2011;6:261–76.

26. Kline JA. Shock. In: Rosen P, Marx J, editors. Emergency medicine; concepts and clinical practice. 5th edition. St Louis (MO): Mosby; 2002. p. 33–47.

27. Shah MR, Hasselblad V, Stevenson LW, et al. Impact of the pulmonary artery catheter in critically ill patients: meta-analysis of randomized clinical trials. JAMA 2005;294:1664–70.

28. Joseph M, Disney P. Transthoracic echocardiography to identify or exclude cardiac cause of shock. Chest 2004;126:1592–7.

29. Bealieu Y. Specific skill set and goals of focused echocardiography for critical care physicians. Crit Care Med 2007;35:S144–9.

30. Grifoni S, Olivotto I, Cecchini P, et al. Utility of an integrated clinical, echocardiographic and venous ultrasound approach for triage of patients with suspected pulmonary embolism. Am J Cardiol 1998;82:1230–5.

31. Viellard-Baron A, Page B, Augarde R, et al. Acute cor pulmonale in massive pulmonary embolism: incidence, echocardiography pattern, clinical implications and recovery rate. Intensive Care Med 2001;27:1481–6.

32. Mookadam F, Jiamsripong P, Goel R, et al. Critical appraisal on the utility of echocardiography in the management of acute pulmonary embolism. Cardiol Rev 2010;18:29–37.

33. Randazzo MR, Snoey ER, Levitt MA, et al. Accuracy of emergency physician assessment of left ventricular ejection fraction and central venous pressure using echocardiography. Acad Emerg Med 2003;10:973–7.

34. Jardin F, Veillard-Baron A. Ultrasonographic examination of the vena cavae. Intensive Care Med 2006;32:203–6.

35. Marik PA. Techniques for assessment of intravascular volume in critically ill patients. J Int Care Med 2009;24(5):329–37.

36. Blehar DJ, Dickman E, Gaspari R. Identification of congestive heart failure via respiratory variation of inferior vena cava. Am J Em Med 2009;27:71–5.

37. Nagdev AD, Merchant RC, Tirado-Gonzalez A, et al. Emergency department bedside ultrasonographic measurement of the caval index for noninvasive determination of low central venous pressure. Ann Emerg Med 2010;55:290–5.

38. Schefold JC, Storm C, Bercker S, et al. Inferior vena cava diameter correlates with invasive hemodynamic measures in mechanically ventilated intensive care patients with sepsis. J Emerg Med 2010;38(5):632–7.

39. Jang T, Aubin C, Naunheim R, et al. Ultrasonography of the internal jugular vein in patients with dyspnea without jugular venous distention on physical examination. Ann Emerg Med 2004;44:160–8.

40. Simon MA, Kliner DE, Girod JP, et al. Detection of elevated right atrial pressure using a simple bedside ultrasound measure. Am Heart J 2010;159:421–7.

41. Connolly JP. Hemodynamic measurements during a tension pneumothorax. Crit Care Med 1993;21:294–6.

42. Carvalho P, Hilderbrandt J, Charan NB. Changes in bronchial and pulmonary arterial blood flow with

progressive tension pneumothorax. J Appl Physiol 1996;81:1664–9.

43. Volpicelli G, Caramello V, Cardinale L, et al. Bedside ultrasound of the lung for the monitoring of acute decompensated heart failure. Am J Em Med 2008;26:585–91.

44. Lichtenstein D. Ultrasound examination of the lungs in the ICU. Pediatr Crit Care 2009;10(6): 693–8.

45. Lensing AW, Prandoni P, Brandjes D, et al. Detection of deep vein thrombosis by real time B-mode ultrasonography. N Engl J Med 1989;320:342–5.

46. Birdwell BG, Raskob GE, Whitsett TL, et al. The clinical validity of normal compression ultrasonography in outpatients suspected of having deep venous thrombosis. Ann Intern Med 1998; 128:1–7.

47. Farahmand S, Farnia M, Shahriaran S, et al. The accuracy of limited B-mode compression technique in diagnosing deep venous thrombosis in lower extremities. Am J Emerg Med 2011;29(6): 687–90.

48. Labovitz AJ, Noble VE, Bierig M. Focused cardiac ultrasound in the emergent setting: a consensus statement of the American Society of Echocardiographers and the American College of Emergency Physicians. J Am Soc Echocardiogr 2010;23(12): 1225–30.

49. Blaivas M. Incidence of pericardial effusions in patients presenting to the emergency department with unexplained dyspnea. Acad Emerg Med 2001;8:1143–6.

50. Shabetai R. Pericardial effusions: haemodynamic spectrum. Heart 2004;90:255–6.

51. Spodick DH. Acute cardiac tamponade. N Engl J Med 2003;349:684–90.

52. Trojanos CA, Porembka DT. Assessment of left ventricular function and hemodynamics with transesophageal echocardiography. Crit Care Clin 1996;12:253–72.

53. Russo AM, O'Connor WH, Waxman HL. Atypical presentations and echocardiographic findings in patients with cardiac tamponade occurring early and late after cardiac surgery. Chest 1993;104: 71–8.

54. Poelaert J, Schmidt C, Colardyn F. Transesophageal echocardiography in the critically ill patient. Anaesthesia 1998;53:55–68.

55. Nabazivadeh SA, Meskshar A. Ultrasonic diagnosis of cardiac tamponade in trauma patients using the collapsibility index of the inferior vena cava. Acad Radiol 2007;14:505–6.

56. Mandavia DP, Hoffner RJ, Mahaney K, et al. Bedside echocardiography by emergency physicians. Ann Emerg Med 2001;38:377–82.

57. Tayal VS, Kline JA. Emergency echocardiography to determine pericardial effusions in patients with PEA and near PEA states. Resuscitation 2003;59: 315–8.

58. Merce J, Sagrista SJ. Correlation between clinical and doppler echocardiographic findings in patients with moderate and large pericardial effusions. Am Heart J 1999;138:759–64.

59. Tsang T, Enriquez-Sarano M, Freeman WK. Consecutive 1127 therapeutic echocardiographically guided pericardiocenteses: clinical profile, practice patterns and outcomes spanning 21 years. Mayo Clin Proc 2002;77:429–36.

60. Amico AF, Lichtenberg GS, Reisner SA, et al. Superiority of visual versus computerized echocardiographic estimation of radionuclide left ventricular ejection fraction. Am Heart J 1989;118:1259–65.

61. Moore CL, Rose GA, Tayal VS, et al. Determination of left ventricular function by emergency physician echocardiography of hypotensive patients. Acad Emerg Med 2002;9:186–93.

62. Picard MH, Davidoff R, Sleeper LA. Echocardiographic predictors of survival and response to early revascularization in cardiogenic shock. Circulation 2003;107:279–84.

63. Reynolds HR, Hochman JS. Cardiogenic shock: current concepts and improving outcomes. Circulation 2008;117:686–97.

64. Jones AE, Craddock PA, Tayal VS, et al. Diagnostic accuracy of identification of left ventricular function among emergency department patients with non-traumatic symptomatic undifferentiated hypotension. Shock 2005;24:513–7.

65. Parker M, Shelhamer J, Baruch S, et al. Profound but reversible myocardial depression in patients with septic shock. Ann Intern Med 1984;100: 483–90.

66. Rivers E, Nguyen B, Haystad S, et al. Early goal directed therapy in the treatment of severe sepsis and septic shock. N Engl J Med 2001; 345:1368–77.

67. Breitkreutz R, Walcher F, Seeger F. Focused echocardiographic evaluation in resuscitation management: concept of an advanced life support-conformed algorithm. Crit Care Med 2007;35(5): S150–61.

68. Hernandez C, Shuler K, Hannan H, et al. C.A.U.S.E.: cardiac arrest ultrasound exam. A better approach to managing patients in primary non-arrythmogenic cardiac arrest. Resuscitation 2008;76:198–206.

69. Breitkreutz R, Price S, Steiger HV, et al. Focused echocardiographic examination in life support and peri-resuscitation of emergency patients: a prospective trial. Resuscitation 2010;81:1527–33.

70. Haas M, Allendorfer J, Walcher F, et al. Focused examination of cerebral blood flow in peri-resuscitation: a new advanced life support compliant concept-an extension of the focused echocardiography

evaluation in life support examination. Crit Ultrasound J 2010;2:1–12.

71. Blaivas M, Fox JC. Outcome in cardiac arrest patients found to have cardiac standstill on bedside emergency department echocardiogram. Acad Emerg Med 2001;8:616–21.

72. Salen P, Melniker L, Choolijan C, et al. Does the presence or absence of sonographically identified cardiac activity predict resuscitation outcomes of cardiac arrest patients? Am J Emerg Med 2005; 23:459–62.

73. Nazeyrollas D, Metz D, Jolly D, et al. Use of transthoracic Doppler echocardiography combined with clinical and electrographic data to predict acute pulmonary embolism. Eur Heart J 1996;17:779–86.

74. Jardin F, Duborg O, Bourdarias JP. Echocardiographic pattern of acute cor pulmonale. Chest 1997;111:209–17.

75. Jardin F, Dubourg O, Gueret P, et al. Quantitative two dimensional echocardiography in massive pulmonary embolism: emphasis on ventricular interdependence and leftward septal displacement. J Am Coll Cardiol 1987;10:1201–6.

76. Madan A, Schwartz C. Echocardiographic visualization of acute pulmonary embolus and thrombolysis in the ED. Am J Emerg Med 2004;22:294–300.

77. Stein J. Opinions regarding the diagnosis and management of venous thrombo-embolic disease. ACCP Consensus Committee on pulmonary embolism. Chest 1996;109:233–7.

78. Rudoni R, Jackson R. Use of two-dimensional echocardiography for the diagnosis of pulmonary embolus. J Emerg Med 1998;16:5–8.

79. Jackson RE, Rudoni RR, Hauser AM, et al. Prospective evaluation of two dimensional transthoracic echocardiography in emergency department patients with suspected pulmonary embolism. Acad Emerg Med 2000;7:994–8.

80. Miniati M, Monti S, Pratali L, et al. Value of transthoracic echocardiography in the diagnosis of pulmonary embolism: results of a prospective study in unselected patients. Am J Med 2001;110(7):528–35.

81. Gifroni S, Olivotto I, Cecchini P, et al. Short term clinical outcome of patients with acute pulmonary embolism, normal blood pressure and echocardiographic right ventricular dysfunction. Circulation 2000;101:2817–22.

82. Becattini C, Agnelli G. Acute pulmonary embolism: risk stratification in the emergency department. Intern Emerg Med 2007;2:119–29.

83. Frazee BW, Snoey ER. Diagnostic role of ED ultrasound in deep venous thrombosis and pulmonary embolism. Am J Emerg Med 1999;17:271–8.

84. Konstantinides S, Geibel A, Heusel G, et al. Heparin plus alteplase compared with heparin alone in patients with submassive pulmonary embolus. N Engl J Med 2002;347:1143–50.

85. Kucher N, Goldhaber SZ. Management of massive pulmonary embolism. Circulation 2005; 112:e28–32.

86. Jaff MR, McMurtry S, Archer S, et al. Management of massive and submassive pulmonary embolism, iliofemoral deep venous thrombosis and chronic thrombo-embolic pulmonary embolism: a scientific statement from the American Heart Association. Circulation 2011;123:1788–830.

87. Wallace DJ, Allison M, Stone MB. Inferior vena cava percentage collapse during resuscitation is affected by the sampling location: an ultrasound study in healthy volunteers. Acad Emerg Med 2010;17:96–9.

88. Kircher B, Himelman R. Noninvasive estimation of right atrial pressure from the inspiratory collapse of the inferior vena cava. Am J Cardiol 1990;66: 493–6.

89. Simonson JS, Schiller NB. Sonospirometry: a new method for noninvasive measurement of mean right atrial pressure based on two dimensional echocardiographic measurements of the inferior vena cava during measured inspiration. J Am Coll Cardiol 1988;11:557–64.

90. Rudski LG, Lai WW, Afilalo J, et al. Guidelines for the echocardiographic assessment of the right heart in adults: a report from the American Society of Echocardiography. J Am Soc Echocardiogr 2010;23:685–713.

91. Barbier C, Loubieres Y, Schmit C, et al. Respiratory changes in inferior vena cava diameter are helpful in predicting fluid responsiveness in ventilated septic patients. Intensive Care Med 2004;30: 1704–46.

92. Lyon M, Blaivas M, Brannam L. Sonographic measurement of the inferior vena cava as a marker of blood loss. Am J Emerg Med 2005;23:45–50.

93. Feissel M, Michard F. The respiratory variation in inferior vena cava diameter as a guide to fluid therapy. Intensive Care Med 2004;30:1834–7.

94. Simon MA, Kliner DE, Girod JP, et al. Detection of elevated right atrial pressure using a simple bedside ultrasound measure. Am Heart J 2010; 159:421–7.

95. Moore CL, Tham ET, Samuels KJ, et al. Tissue doppler of early mitral filling correlates with simulated volume loss in health subjects. Acad Emerg Med 2010;17(11):1162–8.

96. Riley DC, Gerson S, Arbo J. Emergency department right atrial pressure and intravascular volume estimation using right ventricular tissue doppler bedside ultrasonography. Crit Ultrasound J 2010; 2:31–3.

97. Gracias VH, Frankel HL, Gupta R, et al. Defining the learning curve for the Focused Abdominal Sonogram for Trauma (FAST) examination: implications for credentialing. Am Surg 2001;67:364–8.

98. Branney SW, Wolfe RE, Moore EE, et al. Quantitative sensitivity of ultrasound in detecting free intraperitoneal fluid. J Trauma 1995;39:375–80.

99. Von Kuenssberg Jehle D, Stiller G, Wagner D. Sensitivity in detecting free intraperitoneal fluid with the pelvic views of the FAST exam. Am J Emerg Med 2003;21:476–8.

100. Stengel D, Bauwens K, Rademache RG, et al. Association between compliance with methodological standards of diagnostic research and reported test accuracy: meta-analysis of focused assessment of US for trauma. Radiology 2005; 236:102–11.

101. Melniker LA. The value of focused assessment with sonography in trauma examination for the need for operative intervention in blunt torso trauma: a rebuttal to 'emergency ultrasound-based algorithms for diagnosing blunt abdominal trauma (review)' from the Cochrane Collaboration. Crit Ultrasound J 2009;1:73–84.

102. Sisley AC, Rozycki GS, Ballard RB, et al. Rapid detection of traumatic effusion using surgeon-performed ultrasonography. J Trauma 1998;44:291–6.

103. Ma OJ, Mateer JR. Trauma ultrasound examination versus chest radiography in the detection of hemothorax. Ann Emerg Med 1997;29:312–5.

104. Brooks A, Davies B, Smethhurst M, et al. Emergency ultrasound in the acute assessment of haemothorax. Emerg Med J 2004;21:44–6.

105. McEwan K, Thompson P. Ultrasound to detect haemothorax after chest injury. Emerg Med J 2007;24:581–2.

106. Gamblin TC, Wall CE Jr, Rover GM, et al. Delayed splenic rupture: case reports and review of the literature. J Trauma 2005;59:1231–4.

107. Blaivas M. Emergency department paracentesis to determine intraperitoneal fluid identity discovered on bedside ultrasound of unstable patients. J Emerg Med 2005;29:461–5.

108. Subotich D, Mandarich D. Accidentally created tension pneumothorax in patient with primary spontaneous pneumothorax—confirmation of the experimental studies, putting into question the classical explanation. Med Hypotheses 2005;64:170–3.

109. Soldati G, Testa A, Sher S, et al. Occult traumatic pneumothorax: diagnostic accuracy of lung ultrasonography in the emergency department. Chest 2008;133:204–11.

110. Wilkerson RG, Stone MB. Sensitivity of bedside ultrasound and supine anteroposterior chest radiographs for the identification of pneumothorax after blunt trauma. Acad Em Med 2009;17:11–7.

111. Sartori S, Tombesi P, Trevisani L, et al. Accuracy of transthoracic sonography in detection of pneumothorax after sonographically guided lung biopsy: prospective comparison with chest radiography. Am J Roentgenol 2007;188:37–41.

112. Zhang M, Liu ZH, Yang JX, et al. Rapid detection of pneumothorax by ultrasonography in patients with multiple trauma. Crit Care 2006;10:R112.

113. Garofalo G, Busso M, Perotto F, et al. Ultrasound diagnosis of pneumothorax. Radiol Med 2006;11:516–25.

114. Blaivas M, Lyon M, Duggal S. A prospective comparison of supine chest radiography and bedside ultrasound for the diagnosis of traumatic pneumothorax. Acad Emerg Med 2005;12:844–9.

115. Knudtson JL, Dort JM, Helmer SD, et al. Surgeon performed ultrasound for pneumothorax in the trauma suite. J Trauma 2004;56:527–30.

116. Lichtenstein DA, Menu Y. A bedside ultrasound sign ruling out pneumothorax in the critically ill. Lung sliding. Chest 1995;108:1345–8.

117. Slater A, Goodwin M, Anderson KE, et al. COPD can mimic the appearance of pneumothorax on thoracic ultrasound. Chest 2006;129:545–50.

118. Lichtenstein DA, Meziere GA. Relevance of lung ultrasound in the diagnosis of acute respiratory failure: the BLUE protocol. Chest 2008;134:117–25.

119. Blaivas M, Tsung JW. Point-of-care sonographic detection of left endobronchial main stem intubation and obstruction versus endotracheal intubation. J Ultrasound Med 2008;27:785–9.

120. Lichtenstein D, Meziere G, Biderman P, et al. The "lung point": an ultrasound sign specific to pneumothorax. Intensive Care Med 2000;26:1434–40.

121. Lichtenstein D, Meziere G, Biderman P, et al. The comet-tail artifact: an ultrasound sign ruling out pneumothorax. Intensive Care Med 1999;25:383–8.

122. Lichtenstein D, Meziere G, Biderman P, et al. The comet tail artifact: an ultrasound sign of alveolar-interstitial syndrome. Am J of Resp Crit Care Med 1997;156:1640–6.

123. Soldati G, Copetti R, Sher S. Sonographic interstitial syndrome: the sound of lung water. J Ultrasound Med 2009;28:163–74.

124. Agricola E, Bove T, Oppizzi M, et al. "Ultrasound comet-tail images": a marker of pulmonary edema: a comparative study with wedge pressure and extravascular lung water. Chest 2005;127:1690–5.

125. Volpicelli G, Noble VE, Liteplo A, et al. Decreased sensitivity of lung ultrasound limited to the anterior chest in emergency department diagnosis of cardiogenic pulmonary edema: a retrospective analysis. Crit Ultrasound J 2010;2:47–52.

126. Volpicelli G, Caramello V, Cardinale L, et al. Bedside ultrasound of the lung for the monitoring of acute decompensated heart failure. Am J Emerg Med 2008;26:585–91.

127. Rohrer MJ, Cutler BS, Wheeler HB. Long-term survival and quality of life following ruptured abdominal aneurysm. Arch Surg 1988;123:1213–7.

128. Hendrickson RG, Dean AJ, Costantino TG. A novel use of ultrasound in pulseless electrical activity: the

diagnosis of an acute abdominal aortic aneurysm rupture. J Emerg Med 2001;21:141–4.

129. Dent B, Kendall RJ, Boyle AA, et al. Emergency ultrasound of the abdominal aorta by UK emergency physicians: a prospective cohort study. Emerg Med J 2007;24:547–9.

130. Costantino TG, Bruno EC, Handly N, et al. Accuracy of emergency medicine ultrasound in the evaluation of abdominal aortic aneurysm. J Emerg Med 2005;29:455–60.

131. Tayal VS, Graf CD, Gibbs MA. Prospective study of accuracy and outcome of emergency ultrasound for abdominal aortic aneurysm over two years. Acad Emerg Med 2003;10:867–71.

132. Kuhn M, Bonnin RL, Davey MJ, et al. Emergency department ultrasound scanning for abdominal aortic aneurysm: accessible, accurate, and advantageous. Ann Emerg Med 2000;36:219–23.

133. Nevitt MP, Ballard DJ, Hallett JW Jr. Prognosis of abdominal aortic aneurysms. A population-based study. N Engl J Med 1989;321:1009–14.

134. Moore CL, Holliday RS, Hwang JQ, et al. Screening for abdominal aortic aneurysm in asymptomatic at-risk patients using emergency ultrasound. Am J Emerg Med 2008;26:883–7.

135. Kodolitsch Y, Krause N, Spielmann R, et al. Diagnostic potential of combined transthoracic echocardiography and x-ray computed tomography in suspected aortic dissection. Clin Cardiol 1999;22:345–52.

136. Blaivas M, Sierzenski PR. Dissection of the proximal thoracic aorta: a new ultrasonographic sign in the subxiphoid view. Am J Emerg Med 2002;20:344–8.

137. Fojtik JP, Costantino TG, Dean AJ. The diagnosis of aortic dissection by emergency medicine ultrasound. J Emerg Med 2007;32:191–6.

138. Budhram G, Reardon R. Diagnosis of ascending aortic dissection using emergency department bedside echocardiogram. Acad Emerg Med 2008;15:584.

139. Perkins AM, Liteplo A, Noble VE. Ultrasound diagnosis of type A aortic dissection. J Emerg Med 2010;38(4):490–3.

140. Clevert DA, Rupp N, Reiser M, et al. Improved diagnosis of vascular dissection by ultrasound B-flow: a comparison with color-coded Doppler and power Doppler sonography. Eur Radiol 2005;15:342–7.

141. Kearon CK, Julian JA, Math M, et al. Noninvasive diagnosis of deep venous thrombosis. Ann Intern Med 1998;128:663–77.

142. Pezullo JA, Perkins AB, Cronan JJ. Symptomatic deep vein thrombosis: diagnosis with limited compression US. Radiology 1996;198:67–70.

143. Blaivas M. Ultrasound in the detection of venous thromboembolism. Crit Care Med 2007;35(Suppl 5):S224–34.

144. Jolly BT, Massarin E, Pigman EC. Color Doppler ultrasound by emergency physicians for the diagnosis of acute deep venous thrombosis. Acad Emerg Med 1997;4:129–32.

145. Eskandari MK, Sugimoto H, Richardson T, et al. Is color flow duplex a good diagnostic test for detection of isolated calf vein thrombosis in high risk patients? Angiology 2000;51:705–10.

146. Poppiti R, Papinocolau G, Perese S. Limited B-mode venous scanning versus complete color flow duplex venous scanning for detection of proximal deep venous thrombosis. J Vasc Surg 1995;22:553–7.

147. Bernardi E, Camporese G, Buller H, et al. Serial 2 point ultrasonography plus d-dimer vs. whole leg color ceded Doppler ultrasonography for diagnosing suspected symptomatic deep vein thrombosis. JAMA 2008;300:1653–9.

148. Baarslag HJ, Van Beek EJ, Koopman MM. Prospective study of color duplex ultrasonography compared with contrast venography in patients suspected of having deep venous thrombosis of the upper extremities. J Intern Med 2002;136:865–72.

149. Frazee BW, Snoey ER, Levitt A. Emergency department compression ultrasound to diagnose proximal deep vein thrombosis. J Emerg Med 2001;20:107–11.

150. Jang T, Docherty M, Aubin S, et al. Resident performed compression ultrasonography for the detection of proximal deep vein thrombosis: fast and accurate. Acad Emerg Med 2004;11:319–22.

151. Burnside PR, Brown MD, Kline JA. Systematic review of emergency physician- performed ultrasonography for lower-extremity deep vein thrombosis. Acad Emerg Med 2008;15:493–8.

152. Kline JA, O'Malley PM, Tayal VS, et al. Emergency clinician-performed compression ultrasonography for deep venous thrombosis of the lower extremity. Ann Emerg Med 2008;52:437–45.

153. Blaivas M, Lambert MJ, Harwood RA, et al. Lower extremity doppler for deep venous thrombosis: can emergency physicians be accurate and fast? Acad Emerg Med 2000;7:120–6.

154. Rose JS, Bair AE, Mandavia DP. The UHP ultrasound protocol: a novel ultrasound approach to the empiric evaluation of the undifferentiated hypotensive patient. Am J Emerg Med 2001;19:299–302.

Index

Moving?

Make sure your subscription moves with you!

To notify us of your new address, find your **Clinics Account Number** (located on your mailing label above your name), and contact customer service at:

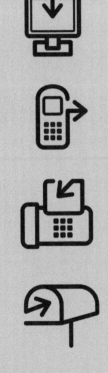

Email: journalscustomerservice-usa@elsevier.com

800-654-2452 (subscribers in the U.S. & Canada)
314-447-8871 (subscribers outside of the U.S. & Canada)

Fax number: 314-447-8029

Elsevier Health Sciences Division
Subscription Customer Service
3251 Riverport Lane
Maryland Heights, MO 63043

ELSEVIER

Printed and bound by CPI Group (UK) Ltd, Croydon, CR0 4YY

03/10/2024

01040357-0003